AF348471

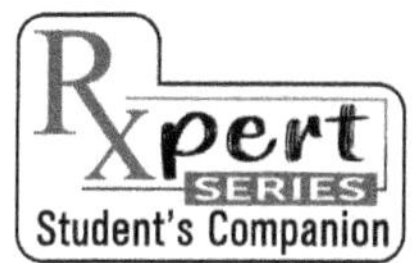

Community Pharmacy and Management

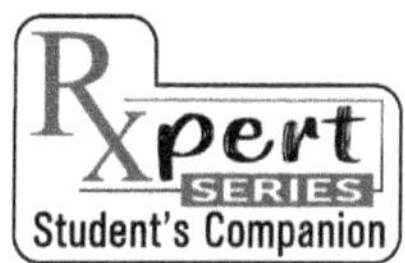

Community Pharmacy and Management

Shiv Kumar Prajapati

Assistant Professor

Pallavi Manish Lavhale

Professor & Principal

Payal Kesharwani

Assistant Professor

Jyoti Chandra

Institute of Pharmacy,
Ram-Eesh Institute of Vocational and Technical Education,
Greater Noida - 201310, U.P.

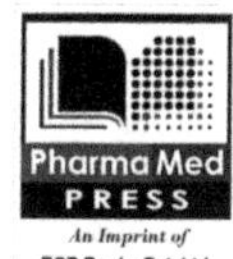

PharmaMed Press

An imprint of BSP Books Pvt. Ltd
4-4-309/316, Giriraj Lane,
Sultan Bazar, Hyderabad - 500 095.

Community Pharmacy and Management
*by Shiv Kumar Prajapati, Pallavi Manish Lavhale, Payal Kesharwani
and Jyoti Chandra*

© 2023, *by Publisher*

Disclaimer: The authors and the publishers have taken due care to provide the authentic, reliable and up to date information related to the subject. However, neither the authors nor the publisher shall be responsible for any liability for any damage caused as a result of use of this book. The respective user must check the accuracy from other sources too.

Published by:

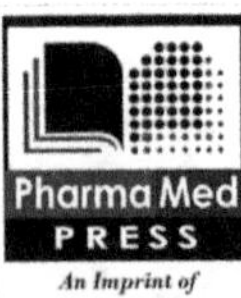

PharmaMed Press

An imprint of BSP Books Pvt. Ltd.
4-4-309/316, Giriraj Lane, Sultan Bazar, Hyderabad - 500 095.
Phone: 040-23445688; Fax: 91+40-23445611
e-mail: info@pharmamedpress.com
www.pharmamedpress.com/pharmamedpress.net

ISBN: 978-93-95039-48-2 (Hardback)

Preface

Health Care needs have gained a lot of public awareness and importance in recent times. The role of Community Pharmacist is well recognized and valued in the Indian Health care system.

This book "Community Pharmacy and Management" has been written as per the new syllabus of Diploma in Pharmacy by the Pharmacy Council of India. An attempt has been made by the authors to provide benefit to the students and the educators of Diploma in Pharmacy. The book covers important topics like Good Pharmacy Practice, Prescription handling, Patient counselling, Medication adherence, Health screening services, OTC medications and Community Pharmacy Management.

The coverage of the topics is comprehensive so that students can use it even for self-study along with short answer questions and long answer questions at the end of each chapter. The authors hope that the book will gain popularity among readers and their criticism and suggestions shall help us in improving the quality of the book for future editions.

- Authors

Contents

Prescription and Prescription Handling

CHAPTER 4

Communications Skills

CHAPTER 5

Patient Counselling

CHAPTER 6

Medication Adherence

CHAPTER 7

Health Screening Services in Community Pharmacy

CHAPTER 8

Over The Counter (OTC) Medications

CHAPTER 9

Community Pharmacy Management

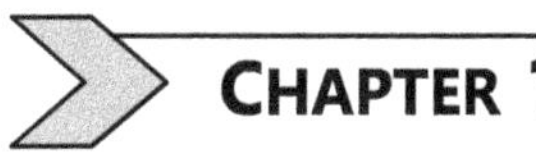

CHAPTER 1

Community Pharmacy Practice

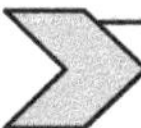

1.1 Introduction

Enjoying the highest possible level of "health" is a fundamental right of all human beings. Health is a comprehensive concept that involves an interdisciplinary team of healthcare providers to provide optimal healthcare to patients. The preamble to WHO's constitution defines "Health as a state of complete physical, mental and social well-being and not merely the absence of disease or infirmity. Community Pharmacy practice takes place in a medical setting and exists to benefit both individual patients as well as society by improving patient's quality of life.

Definition

Community Pharmacy includes all privately owned facilities and is responsible for serving society to meet the needs of medicines and pharmaceutical services. "Community Pharmacy is defined as a place where the medicines are stocked and dispensed to the patients on a valid prescription".

The main responsibilities of a community pharmacy include compounding, counseling, and dispensing of drugs to the patients with care, accuracy, and legality along with the proper procurement, storage, dispensing and documentation of medicines.

Community pharmacists are health care professionals who are available to the public and dispense drugs by prescription or over-the-counter where permitted legally.

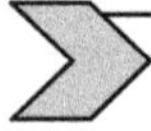

1.2   History and Development of Community Pharmacy

The emergence of community pharmacies in India can be traced back to British India, where symptomatic drugs were introduced in the late 19th century and became available through drug stores. In the course of colonial period, the pharmacy profession was more business-oriented, and those who were trained to sell drugs were referred to as drug sellers or, in some cases, dispensers. The prescribing and dispensing functions were traditionally performed by the physicians/doctors or sometimes by their assistants called "Compounders". When India gained independence in 1947, it inherited an unorganized system for the pharmacy profession from the British rulers, and there were no legal restrictions on the practice of pharmacy. The concept of pharmacy practice did not emerge until after independence. Earlier in the century, anyone could prepare any drug in any way and give it to a patient without being held responsible for it. The Pharmacy Act came into force in 1948 as the nation's first minimum educational qualification standards for pharmacy in order to correct this state of affairs and regulate pharmacy practice, education, and profession.

After the enactment of the Pharmacy Act 1948, pharmacists working in India are required to have a pharmacist registration certificate issued by the state in which they wish to practice. For obtaining registration certificate, a prospective pharmacist must obtain a diploma (D. Pharm.) from a Pharmacy Council of India-accredited pharmacy institute. D. Pharm. and B. Pharm. holders are both permitted to practice in pharmacy sector. Most of the community pharmacies now are managed by the individuals who are D. Pharm. holders (diploma pharmacists). The D. Pharm. requires at least two years of study, as well as 500 hours of practical training spread over three months in a hospital or community pharmacy. Prior to 1984, a person without a pharmacist degree could be registered as a pharmacist in the first register of the Pharmacy Act having five years of experience in compounding and dispensing medicines in hospitals or clinics. The provisions of Article 32B of the pharmacy act(related to displaced persons or repatriates) were abused in the 1980s, and many uneducated and untrained people registered their names as pharmacists (called non-diploma pharmacist).

1.2.1   International Scenario

The profession of pharmacists has changed significantly in the last few decades. The focus has been shifted from the product to the patient. The role of pharmacists has evolved from drug commanders and suppliers to service and information providers and ultimately to patient care providers through drug supply services.

In order to meet the professional challenges and gain recognition as a health care professional. community pharmacists in developed countries like Australia, United States, and United Kingdom are embracing the new professional responsibilities in addition to dispensing. They have also given pharmacists prescription rights in order to reduce the burden on physicians and improve the quality of care. However, in comparison to the Western world, the role of the community pharmacist in India is limited. New responsibilities for community pharmacists include reviewing medication records, providing advice on medication use, un-biased drug information, medication reviews, health care services, and providing education on smoking cessation and family planning.

In Australia, the principle activity of community pharmacy is the distribution of medicines under the pharmaceutical benefits scheme (PBS), to the citizens. Community pharmacists in Australia provides a wide range of services, including home medication reviews, population screening and testing for hypertension, glaucoma, and diabetes, in addition to providing necessary patient counselling on drugs and diseases.

In United Kingdom, pharmacists are involved in public health education programs about medication safety, dental health, coronary disease prevention, and patient compliance, using posters, leaflets, badges, and audiovisual displays as information sources. In addition to traditional roles dispensing medicines community pharmacist are also engaging themselves in community services to allow better working and integration.

Pharmacists in United States are trained pharmaceutical professionals who use their knowledge to improve the health of their patients. Responsibilities include dosing, ensuring the safety and appropriateness of prescribed treatments, and monitoring patient health and progression.

1.2.2 Indian Scenario

In terms of pharmaceutical production, exports, and imports, India ranks among the top fifteen countries in the world. This is encouraging, but in India, pharmacy is merely a technically oriented job of preparing and dispensing drugs. The country has approximately 800000 retail pharmacies. The majority of them are concentrated in urban areas. Those which have the facility of compounding are permitted to use the term pharmacy while others are permitted to be called as either a chemist and druggist or medical store. The legal requirements for opening a pharmacy under Article 42 of the Drugs and Cosmetics Act require a qualified person or a "registered pharmacist" and all dispensing activities must be carried out in the presence of the pharmacist. Unfortunately, in many of them a pharmacist is not present all the times.

In India, the minimum qualification for registration as a "pharmacist" is a pharmacy diploma (D.Pharm), but in most developed countries, the minimum qualification for registration is B.Pharm or Pharm D. Only the pharmacist should be permitted to dispense medications under strict legal restrictions. A vast majority of the medical stores/pharmacies are owned by independents. In the last 10 years some Indian chains and online pharmacies have emerged and are posing tough competitions to independents. The concept and technique of compounding prescription has already been wiped out in the last 30 years, and today only 1% of prescriptions are compounded. The regional (retail) pharmacy sector is the primary source of medicine for both outpatients and inpatients. The most common activity performed at a pharmacy is to fill out a prescription. In many cases, prescription filling is basically done by people who are not qualified and who view pharmacy profession as a trade.

Listed below are the problems which are faced by community pharmacies are:

1. Inadequate incentives and profit margin

2. Overcrowding of urban and suburban community pharmacies in co-located areas is the reason for unhealthy competition and lack of professional conceptual development in the realm of practice.

3. Anyone can open a pharmacy. It is not an exclusive domain of the pharmacist

4. Professional fee- at present in India, there is no practice of charging professional fee for dispensing medicine

Despite numerous obstacles, community pharmacy services are central to the safe and effective management of medicines for the health promotion and advancement. With rapid changes in health care delivery and rising patient expectations, community pharmacies are expected to change accordingly.

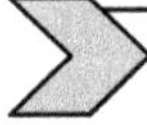 **Exercise Questions**

Multiple Choice Questions

1. As per WHO.........................is a state of complete physical, mental and social well-being and not merely the absence of disease or infirmity

   a. Health   b. Happiness

   c. Gentle   d. Lethargy

2. Community Pharmacy is defined as a place where the medicines are ....to the patients on a valid prescription"

    a.   Stocked
    b.   Dispensed
    c.   Both a & b
    d.   None of the above

3. In India, the minimum qualification for registration as a "pharmacist" is?

    a.   D.Pharm
    b.   B.Pharm
    c.   Pharm.D
    d.   All the above

4. .... Act came into force in 1948 as the nation's first minimum educational qualification standards for pharmacy

    a.   Drug and Cosmetic Act
    b.   Pharmacy Act
    c.   Drug and Magic Remedies Act
    d.   None of the above

5. The legal requirements for opening a pharmacy under ....of the Drugs and Cosmetics Act require a qualified person or a "registered pharmacist"

    a.   Article 40
    b.   Article 41
    c.   Article 42
    d.   All the above

Answers

    1.   a
    2.   c
    3.   a
    4.   b
    5.   c

Short Answer Questions

1. Write a short on community pharmacy

2. Write a brief descriptive note on the development of community pharmacy

3. Write a short note on international scenario of community pharmacy

Long Answer Questions

1. What do you mean by community pharmacy? Write a detailed note on history and development of community pharmacy in India

2. Write a detailed note on International and Indian scenario of community pharmacy

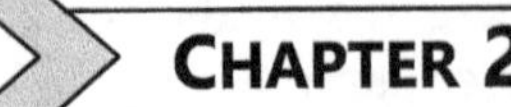 ## CHAPTER 2

Responsibilities of Community Pharmacist and Good Pharmacy Practice

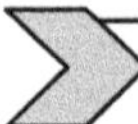 ## 2.1 Introduction

Public health is the basis of the well-being and welfare of all people. Barriers to health include below par access to quality health equipment, trained health care workers and care, insufficient health care workers, exorbitant care costs and include inadequate standards of training for healthcare professionals. Pharmacists, as health-care professionals, play a key role in boosting access to health care. Pharmacists are trained medical professionals who are engaged in the distribution of medicines and are committed to making reasonable efforts to ensure safe and effective use. To meet these drug-related needs, pharmacists are taking on more responsibility for the consequences of drug use and evolving their practices to deliver patients with improved drug-use services.

After completing this chapter, students will be able to understand

♦ Public health and pharmaceutical care

♦ Professional roles of community pharmacists

♦ Good pharmacy practices and standard operating procedures

Pharmaceutical care is an evolutionary and innovative way to practice pharmacies. We need to completely rethink how the pharmacists have worked traditionally. While some pharmacists confuse pharmaceutical care with patient counseling and illness management, pharmaceutical care is much more complex and presents even more challenges and opportunities. The pharmacist must be responsible for preventing and resolving drug-related problems and optimizing drug therapy. It does not end when the patient walks out of the pharmacy. Assessment (understanding of a patient's illness and treatment plan), monitoring, care, documentation, and follow-up are integral parts of pharmaceutical care.

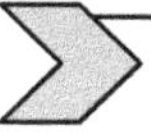 2.2 Roles and Responsibilities of Community Pharmacist

Community pharmacists are an essential component of primary health care and are the most accessible health professionals to the general public. The role of community pharmacists is growing worldwide.

The World Health Organization and the International Federation of Pharmaceuticals have listed the following professional duties for pharmacists:

- Prescription processing
- Dispensing
- Patient counselling
- Drug information services
- Health promotion
- Health screening services
- Responding to symptoms of minor ailments
- Consultation to general practitioners

2.2.1 Prescription Processing

It is expected from the community pharmacist that he should review and check the prescription for its legality, adequacy and potential drug related issues. The pharmacist should dispense the medicines to the patient only upon the satisfaction of the content.

2.2.2 Dispensing

Previously, pharmacists were involved in compounding; however, prepackaged medicines in various dosage forms are now available on the market, making compounding and dispensing obsolete. Therefore, the pharmacist must label the patient's name, age, gender, drug name, medication precautions, prescribing doctor's name, and pharmacy stamp on each item prescribed on the prescription.

2.2.3 Patient Counselling

The majority of patients may not have the right idea about the correct use of the drug because of very brief information provided to them by the physician due to their busy schedule and over patient load. Thus it is the responsibility of pharmacist to educate and inform the clients about the proper use of medications and other health care products.

The pharmacist should counsel the patient or patient's representative in layman language regarding the appropriate use of medicine and maintaining healthy diet and lifestyle in controlling the disease symptoms.

2.2.4   Drug Information Services

A drug information service is a specialized service offered by pharmacists to improve drug knowledge, enable rational prescribing, and reduce medication errors. The main goal of drug information services is to improve patient care by providing an unbiased information on drug issues. A drug information service is an entity or staff dedicated to providing written or oral information about drugs and drug therapies at the request of another healthcare professional, organization, committee, or patient. For providing information on drugs pharmacist may use several primary sources such as peer reviewed journals like LANCET, BMJ etc. or various secondary sources from the databases like IDIS, MicroMedex etc.

2.2.5   Health Promotion

Community pharmacists should be able to educate individuals about healthy habits and lifestyles by organizing various health promotion activities and campaigns such as smoking cessation program, family planning, vaccinations, etc.

2.2.6   Health Screening Services

Health screening services are patient care services provided in community pharmacies by pharmacists that aid in the early detection of disease so that patients can receive treatment as soon as possible. Health screening services helps community pharmacists in assisting and monitoring to manage the chronic diseases such as hypertension, diabetes, and asthma. This will reduce the burden on both the individual and society.

2.2.7   Responding to Symptoms of Minor Ailments

Pharmacists as easily accessible health care professional should be able to provide appropriate medicines to relieve the symptoms of mild illnesses such as colds, diarrhea, body aches, and cramps.

2.2.8   Consultation to General Physician

Comprehensive treatment can improve patient health. This creates an urgent need for interdisciplinary partnerships in the medical community. Optimal pharmacological treatment is critical for achieving therapeutic goals. Professional cooperation between doctors and pharmacists is necessary to ensure good quality of care. Their complementary knowledge and experience can lead to improved health outcomes and reduced treatment costs.

The pharmacist can refer the patient to a general practitioner for proper treatment of the condition. If necessary, the pharmacist will provide the doctor with information about the medicine and emergency medicine to achieve better treatment results.

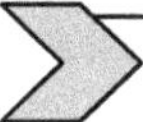 ## 2.3   Good Pharmacy Practices

Good Pharmacy Practice (GPP) is an international standard for pharmaceutical services and was established in 1992 by the World Health Organization (WHO) and the International Federation of Pharmacists (FIP). The GPP component has been further improved and approved by WHO in 1996 to encourage pharmaceutical organizations in each country to attract pharmacists' attention in the field of community pharmacies and hospital pharmacies to evolve the elements of the services they provide to reflect changing conditions.

Definition

Jointly, the WHO and FIP defined "GPP is the practice of pharmacy that responds to the needs of the people who use the pharmacists' services to provide optimal, evidence-based care. To support this practice, it is essential that there be an established national framework of quality standards and guidelines".

2.3.1   Requirements of Good Pharmacy Practice

1. GPP requires that the pharmacist's primary concern in all situations is patient's well-being.
2. GPP requires that the core of pharmacy operations is to assist patients to get the most out of their medications. Its basic functions include the supply of quality-guaranteed medicines and other healthcare products, the provision of appropriate information and advice to patients, the administration of medicines as needed, and monitoring the impact of drug use.
3. GPP requires that the pharmacist's contribution include the promotion of rational and cost-effective prescribing as well as dispensing.
4. GPP requires that the purpose of each element of Pharmacy Service is patient-related, well-defined and effectively communicated to all stakeholders. The key to successfully improving patient safety is multidisciplinary collaboration among health-care professionals.

As per WHO and FIP, GPP requires establishment of certain criteria and standards at the national or appropriate (e.g. state or provincial) level which includes

- **A legal framework that**
  1. States who can practice pharmacy
  2. States the scope of pharmacy practice
  3. Ensures the integrity of the supply chain and the quality of medicines.

- **A workforce framework that**
  1. Ensures the competence of pharmacy staff through continuing professional development (CPD or continuing education (CE)) programmes
  2. Defines the personnel resources needed to provide GPP. 317

- **An economic framework that**
  1. Provides sufficient resources and incentives that are effectively used to ensure the activities undertaken in GPP.

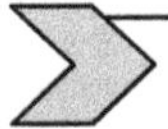

2.4 Standard Operating Procedures

An important aspect of a quality system is that it works according to a well-defined standard operating procedure (SOP). A standard operating procedure is a set of written instructions that describes the step-by-step process that must be followed to perform a routine activity correctly.

2.4.1 Pharmacy Premises

The pharmacy should be located at a place where it can be easily identifiable to the public. The pharmacy's premises should be neat and clean. The word "PHARMACY" should be clearly written in both English and the local language(s) of the area on the façade. People using strollers, wheelchairs, etc. should have easy access to the pharmacy. Pharmaceutical services and products should be provided in a separate area from other activities/services and products. Pharmacists should be easily approachable to the general public for information, advice, and counselling etc. because:

1. Patients may be reluctant or uncomfortable to share about their conditions or medications with a pharmacist if they feel that others may hear their conversation.

2. If the patient's problem/question requires time more than 10 minutes than it requires a space where the patient can sit comfortably.

3. Demonstration of a particular device / diagnostic kit / self-use device using diagrams and videos should be done in an un-disturbed or relevant location.

2.4.1.1 Requirements of Ideal Pharmacy Premises

1. It should be free from rodents, insects and pest

2. The pharmacy should have an uninterrupted supply of energy, particularly for the refrigerator

3. It is desirable to provide drinking water facility to patients and staff

4. There should be enough room for customers to stand comfortably at the service counter, if possible, to sit comfortably while waiting.

5. A sufficient space for displaying information, including pamphlets / materials

6. A separate space known as "counselling Area" for patient counselling, storage of reference resources (e.g. books, internet access etc.) should also be there with additional space for compounding for making extemporaneous preparations

7. Separate waste collection baskets/boxes should be provided to both staff and customers

Excessive light and heat should be avoided in the product storage area. To prevent deterioration of various medicines stored at room temperature, the pharmacy's ambient temperature should be kept within the specified range.

2.4.2 Furniture and Fixtures

Neat, well-placed shelves should be available in the pharmacy for the storage of medicines and other items in order to protect from dust, moisture, and excessive light. Adequate provisions should be made for storing various medicines at the prescribed temperatures.

The counselling area must contain the following

1. A table

2. Chair for pharmacist and patients

3. Cabinets for storing patient's medication records

2.4.3 Equipment

The pharmacy must contain refrigerated storage facilities for the products requiring cold storage temperature

Requirements for counselling area are

1. Reference material

2. Demonstration charts, kits and other material

3. Patient Information leaflets

4. Some basic instruments e.g. Sphygmomanometer, glucometer, stethoscope, etc.

5. Weight and height scale

The pharmacy should have computers with appropriate software for managing various tasks such as

1. Inventory control

2. Billing

3. Generation of timely warning for expiring medicines

4. Patients medication record maintenance

2.4.4 Personnel

All professional activities and operations in community pharmacies are carried out as per the documented guidelines under the supervision of the chief pharmacist. There should be a staff training policy for staff working in the pharmacy including newly recruited staff. Each employee should have defined responsibilities that should be carried out in accordance with documented standard operating procedures.

The pharmacists at the pharmacy should always wear the proper apron / coat and a badge that clearly shows their name and the word "pharmacist."In addition, recent photos, credentials, and registration certificate from the State Pharmacy Council may be prominently displayed for customers entering the pharmacy.

Requirements of pharmacist working in the community pharmacy are:

1. He/she should be a graduate in pharmacy or holding diploma in pharmacy

2. He/she should be registered with state pharmacy council in which they are working

3. Must have completed practical training at community pharmacy

4. Must have completed house training as per organization's staff training policy

5. Should have effective communication skills

6. The pharmacist working in the community pharmacy should be professionally competent so that he/she can assess the prescription and advise the patients regarding selection and appropriate use of drug and OTC medications, drug interactions and adverse drug reaction

7. He/she should be able to evaluate the patient's condition and determine when to refer him or her to a doctor.

2.4.5 Systems

Each operation performed in the pharmacy should have well-defined and documented systems for the proper functioning of community pharmacy.

2.4.5.1 Quality Policy

Quality goals stem from the stated quality policy and are the targets that are set and can be achieved within a specified time frame. Different quality objectives must be established in the pharmacy's various operational areas.

The pharmacy should have a well-documented quality manual that describes the steps that must be taken in order to meet the desired quality goals. The manual should also contain information about the activities, routines, task divisions, work processes, and instructions needed to achieve quality goals in the pharmacy's day-to-day operations. Quality manuals should be available to pharmacy staff for easy reference.

The Chief Pharmacist is responsible for ensuring that the quality policy and quality goals are understood, implemented, and maintained throughout the pharmacy's operations. Audits should be performed on a regular basis to ensure that the pharmacy is meeting its quality goals, and the results should be documented for future review to further improve the process.

2.4.5.2 Service Policy

The pharmacy should have a well-documented service policy that clearly states the nature of services provided in the pharmacy in accordance with its client servicing goals. The nature and level of attention to be given to clients should be addressed in the service policy statement. The service manual should detail the steps that must be taken to provide each service offered by the pharmacy.

2.4.5.3 Staff Training Policy

A well-written and implemented training policy, as well as adequate availability of reference resources such as books, current periodicals, and software, are required to shape the future of community pharmacy.

The pharmacy's evolving out-of-service policy should be incorporated into the training policy. The training policy requires that all pharmacy staff be kept up to date with the development of the area. The training policy should focus on improving communication and interpersonal skills.

The policy should specify the minimum continuing education levels that each staff member must meet in order to achieve the ultimate goal of Pharmaceutical Care. All pharmacy personnel should be trained and be aware of the pharmacy's Quality Policy. They should also be aware of personal hygiene, storage and handling hygiene levels that must be maintained.

The staff training policy must include following in regards to training of pharmacist and pharmacy assistants:

1. For Pharmacist:

    (i)   Communication and counselling skills

    (ii)   Prescription handling

    (iii)   Continuing education on illness

    (iv)   Recent development in pharmacy field

    (v)   Assessing and evaluating "when to refer" to a doctor

2. For Pharmacy Assistants:
   (i)   Communication skills and salesmanship
   (ii) Prescription handling
   (iii) Dispensing, procurement and storage of drugs
   (iv) Assessing and evaluating "when to refer" to a doctor

The policies and procedures for providing education and training should be well documented, regularly reviewed and implemented according to an established schedule. Pharmacists should be encouraged to update their knowledge through scientific literature, textbooks, journals, periodicals, workshops and more. Need to promote networking with pharmacists in other pharmacies

2.4.5.4 Complaint Policy

Pharmacies must set up the grievances redressal policy for all types of oral or written complaints. This should be checked periodically. All complaints need to be dealt with immediately by the pharmacist and appropriate measures must be taken to change the situation.

The nature of the complaint, the name of the wrongdoer, and the action taken must all be documented in a complaint register. The event should be reviewed and evaluated to determine the root cause (s).

2.4.5.5 Drug Recall Policy

The substandard medicines should be recall state-wide or nation –wide immediately and pharmacist should show their active participation in the process. The pharmacist should immediately record all such events after receiving authentic information and alarms. The beginning, progress, and conclusion of the recall should all be thoroughly documented. To detect recall alerts from both regulatory sources and pharmaceutical companies, adequate vigilance must be maintained. In the event of a suspicion, the pharmacist should take immediate action to stop the sale of the drug and notify the appropriate parties.

2.4.5.6 Audit Policy

Audit is performed to ensure and determine that the quality management system is functioning properly and that the intended goals of the pharmacy have been achieved in accordance with the guidelines set out in the Quality Manual. Quality auditing helps the Chief Pharmacist in evaluating the various routine processes and quality systems in the pharmacy. To initiate necessary improvements in community pharmacy set ups, a frequent internal audit and a periodic external audits are required.

The chief pharmacist, along with senior staff or members who have been trained for the purpose, can conduct the internal audit. Internal audits may be performed once every six months, but external audits must be performed at least once a year by external auditors.

All audit procedures must be properly documented. The audit report should be used to identify system flaws and defects so that corrective action can be taken.

2.4.5.7   Documentation System

For achieving and maintaining quality within community pharmacy settings, documentation is a critical activity which needs to be performed on a regular basis. The chief pharmacist is ultimately responsible for documentation.

All required legal documents (regulatory licenses, registrations, permits, etc.) and operational documents (e.g. purchases, invoices, etc. must be properly maintained; legally required records can be displayed by pharmacies while operational records can be archived as required by law. In either cases, they should always be easily accessible when needed.

List of necessary documents required to be maintained

1. Protocols
2. Standard working procedures
3. Operation instructions
4. Quality manual
5. Cleaning and maintenance processes and records
6. Complaint records
7. Audit records (internal & external)
8. Policy documents
9. Personnel details

Furthermore, the documents required for the pharmaceutical care process must be properly maintained and stored which may include

1. Patients' health profile
2. Patients' medication records
3. Records of counselling follow-ups, etc.

2.4.6 Process Guidelines

A socially and economically effective and acceptable operational system should be maintained by a community pharmacy to ensure optimal health and cost effective benefits to the customers.

2.4.6.1 Procurement and Inventory Management

It is the responsibility of pharmacist to check the purchased medicines and other items should meet the standards and legal requirements laid down in the law. Also the chief pharmacist has the additional responsibility of protecting the interests of customers and pharmacies from being fooled by substandard supplies. A proper documented record of the vendor's details (for example, their addresses, contact numbers, names and addresses of their management, technical, and administrative personnel, and copies of various licenses held by them), should be kept in the pharmacy. The pharmacy's designated responsible person(s) should visit the vendor's premises on a regular basis to conduct audits of their premises and systems that are likely to affect the quality of the products. If there are reasons to believe that the vendors are engaging in deliberate, dubious behavior, the chief pharmacist may consider informing the regulatory authorities (s).

Ideal practice for procurement may include the following:

1. Storing the products manufactured by reputed companies
2. Maintaining a 'products list' where all items 'approved' by the pharmacy for stocking
3. Update and review the product list on regular basis (review must be carried out chief pharmacist if any new items are added in the list)
4. Cost effective or economic purchasing should be done for obtaining optimal financial gain for the pharmacy
5. All products received from the supplier must be checked against the invoice to ensure the accuracy of the quality, price, lot number, and expiration date.
6. Any discrepancies should be brought to the supplier's attention for appropriate remedies. All such corrections should be documented and authenticated by an authorized vendor representative.

2.4.6.2 Storage

Before checking for quality, batch number, expiry, and integrity, purchased products should be kept in a separate area of the pharmacy. They should be transferred to their respective storage location after any necessary checks. The product should be stored at ambient temperature and humidity conditions protected from excessive light and dust. Drugs required to be stored in cold temperature should be stored in the refrigerators. For storing the drugs and other items shelves or racks can be used, which should be clean following cleaning schedules and SOPs. Special care should be taken in case of Narcotic Drugs and Psycotropic Substances, and must be kept under lock and key. Shelves should be checked on a regular basis to ensure that drugs with an expiry date approaching are removed. Products near expiry either needs to be stored separately or disposed of. Drugs that have passed the expiration date must be stored separately on locked shelves. With a label "Expired Goods Not For Sale".

2.4.7 Prescription Handling

a) After prescription receiving, the Pharmacist must confirm:
1. Identity of the client
2. Whether the prescription is presented by the client himself or by someone on the client's behalf.

b) The pharmacist should review the prescription for:
1. Therapeutic aspects (Pharmaceutical and pharmacological)
2. Appropriate for an individual
3. Social, legal & economic aspects
4. Legality & completeness of prescription

c) Prescription should be complete in terms of:
1. Name of the Doctor, his /her address and registration number.
2. Name, address, age, sex of the patient
3. Name(s) of the medicine(s), potency, dosage, total amount of the medicines to be supplied.
4. Instruction to the patient
5. Refill information if any
6. Prescribed doctors' signature.

d) Correctness of the prescribed medicine and should be checked for:
1. Dosage
2. Double medication
3. Drug interaction
4. Contraindication
5. History of drug overuse, underuse or misuse

2.4.7.1 Dispensing

2.4.7.1.1 Filling of Prescription

After receiving the prescription pharmacist should start collecting the medicine from the storage area and keep them at the counter for counting and invoicing. The pharmacist should make a final review of prescription for the correctness of prescribed medicines. Appropriate counselling of patient should be done by the pharmacist while dispensing the medicine. Pharmaceuticals need to be properly packaged in order to maintain their integrity. Medicines requiring special care for e.g. vaccines and other biological products which need to be store at cold temperature, should be packed in ice packs to avoid their deterioration and maintaining their integrity at an optimum temperature.

2.4.7.1.2 Extemporaneous Preparations

When preparing extemporaneous preparations, the pharmacist should keep standard operating procedures and standard formulations in mind for his/her reference. To perform any compounding activity methodically, the proposed adjuvants, their quantities, and method of preparation must be written down. Proper documentation of the step-by-step procedure is recommended. The compounding should be done in a neat and clean preparation are using ingredients of pharmaceutical grade or higher. All instruments must be calibrated on a regular basis.

After filling the preparation, the container should be properly labelled with name of the prescription, date of preparation and expiry, patient's name, direction regarding use, quantity, storage and name of the pharmacy.

2.4.8   Counselling and Information for Patient

The welfare of the client is the primary concern of community pharmacists. It is the responsibility of pharmacist to educate and inform the clients about the proper use of medications and other health care products. The pharmacist should assist the client in making decisions about self-care.

The goal of consultation is to achieve the highest level of compliance possible. In order to raise the client's awareness level, pharmacists should provide both oral and written information regarding various illnesses, medicines, and other health care products. In case of doubts or reasons to believe that it would be in the client's best interests to see a doctor or another health care provider as soon as possible, pharmacist must advise the client to do so.

While dispensing medicines to the patients, the pharmacist should check the container should be properly labelled and provided information & advice should be correct, explicit and understandable to the client. To improve the patient's life, the pharmacist must devise strategies for professional counselling on the best use of medications.

At the time of dispensing, the following should be explained to the patient:

1. How to take medication and for how long?
2. When to take medication (e.g. before and after meal)
3. Foods/beverages/tasks need to avoid during therapy.
4. Side effects and precautions during medication
5. What to do in case of skipped dose

2.4.8.1   Patient's Follow-up

Many patients, particularly those with chronic conditions, require continuity of care. Pharmacists should keep track of medications taken by such patients and update the patient's medication history on a regular basis as long as the patient is under their care.

The pharmacist is responsible for making follow-up phone calls or meetings to inquire about the patient's condition and response to the medication, adverse events experienced by the patient, dose and frequency of the medication, and skipped dose (if any).

Possible causes of patient non-compliance should be assessed and counselling should be done accordingly. The pharmacist should inform the patient's physician about all adverse events reported by the patient, along-with all possible reason for patient's non-compliance.

2.4.8.2   Self-care

It is recommended that community pharmacy should have a clear defined health promotion policy. The community pharmacist should encourage the patient about self-care routine and healthy lifestyle which can be done by running health promotion programs and campaigns. The pharmacist should educate and counsel the patient regarding misuse and abuse of drugs and medicine, avoiding alcohol and tobacco etc.

In the event that preventive measures fail or the patient's condition is not serious, the pharmacist may encourage self-medication or suggest non-prescription medications. If the Pharmacist is unsure about the patient's condition, he or she must refer the patient to a doctor. If the patient feels worse or the symptoms do not go away and persists for more than three days even after taking non-prescription medication, than it is the responsibility of the pharmacist that he/she should refer the patient to a doctor. Pharmacies need to develop protocols for self-medication advice and offering non-prescription medicine. The pharmacy should keep a record of all such patients, as well as the advice and medications they receive.

2.4.9 Medication Record

There should be a patient medication record system either manual or computerized so that patient's health and medication history can be assessed as and when required.

The following conditions may necessitate a review of the patient's medication history:

I. If the patient has a chronic disease

II. If certain value or conditions are need to monitor and control for the patient

The most common forms of patient medication records should include the following:

a) All drugs consumed in the previous year or more (drug name, potency, dose taken, length of time taken)

b) Is there a history of allergies or hypersensitivity to any medicine(s)?

c) The patient experienced adverse drug reactions and drug interactions.

d) What medication, if any, was administered to treat the reaction?

e) Does patient have a drug or medicine addiction? Is this known to the prescriber?

f) Is the patient a regular user of alcoholic beverages, tobacco, tea, or coffee? (frequency and amount may be recorded)

g) Does patient have any problems with the medication? Difficulty swallowing, etc.

h) Professional advice provided from time to time.

All patient-related data and information must be kept confidential, stored and maintained so that only authorized persons can access it. Such data can usually be shared with other medical professionals at the patient's explicit request or in the best interests of the patient.

2.4.10   Health Promotion and Ill Health Prevention

According to the World Health Organization (WHO), health promotion is "the process of enabling people to increase control over, and improve, their health". The chief pharmacist must be aware of national policies and various health programs. Pharmacies should actively participate in local and national health promotion campaigns and programs. Continuing education programs and regular interactions with other healthcare providers should be done on a regular basis in order to train the staff involved in health promotion campaigns. Pharmacies should be able to provide advice on several issues, including diabetes, high blood pressure, arthritis, AIDS, breastfeeding, assistive device use, and appropriate medication use.

2.4.11   Pharmacovigilance

During an active conversation with the patient, the pharmacist should be alert to the occurrence of expected and unexpected adverse effects of the medicines. It is the responsibility of pharmacist to maintain the record of adverse effect reported by patient and should provide the patient appropriate instructions to reduce the adverse effects in future, such as advising patient regarding proper use of medication, how and when to use the medicine correctly, food and activities to avoid during medication.

2.4.12   Enhancement of Professional Role and Interaction

Pharmacists must keep abreast of the development of their profession. Good communication skills are required to work closely with other healthcare providers and share what they learn. Pharmacists must maintain positive relationships with other health-care providers.

In the event of a prescription discrepancy the pharmacist should contact the doctor in order to clear his/her doubt in a friendly manner. Before contacting the doctor, the pharmacist should reconfirm that your prescription is incorrect or inconsistent and come up with alternatives / solutions that can be quickly suggested on inquiry from the doctor.

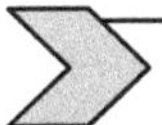

Exercise Questions

Multiple Choice Questions

1. As per WHO & FIP, the professional responsibilities of pharmacists includes;
   a.   Prescription processing& Dispensing
   b.   Health screening services
   c.   Drug information services
   d.   All the above

2. ....is a specialized service offered by pharmacists to improve drug knowledge, enable rational prescribing, and reduce medication errors.
   a.   Patient counseling   b.   Drug information services
   c.   Health screening services   d.   None of the above

3. A ....is a set of written instructions that describes the step-by-step process that must be followed to perform a routine activity correctly
   a.   Standard operating procedures
   b.   Good pharmacy practice
   c.   Both a & b
   d.   None of the above

4. The goal of consultation is to achieve
   a.   Highest patient compliance
   b.   Awareness
   c.   Information on illness and medicines use
   d.   All the above

5. ....is "the process of enabling people to increase control over, and improve, their health"

    a.   Health awareness   b.   Health screening

    c.   Health promotion   d.   None of the above

6. .... Helps in assessing the health and medication history of patient

    a.   Medication record   b.   Patient's health profile

    c.   Personnel details   d.   All the above

Answers

1.	a	2.	b
3.	a	4.	d
5.	c	6.	a

Short Answer Questions

1. Describe the role of community pharmacist in Drug Information Service

2. Write a short note on quality policy of community pharmacy

3. What do you mean by *GPP*? Write the requirement for *GPP*

4. What is patient medication record? Why it is needed?

5. Who is community pharmacist? Write a brief note on the role and responsibilities of community pharmacist in health promotion and health screening service

Long Answer Questions

1. Explain in detail about the role and responsibilities of community pharmacist

2. What do you mean by Standard Operating Procedure? Write a detailed note on SOPs required for prescription handling

3. Write a descriptive note on the personnel requirements for community pharmacy

4. Write a detail note on various policies of a community pharmacy

5. What do you mean by process guidelines? What is the ideal practice for procurement in community pharmacy setting?

6. Write a detailed note on the role of community pharmacist in health promotion and pharmacovigilance.

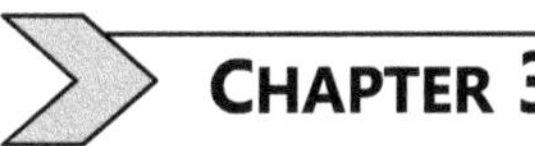

CHAPTER 3

Prescription and Prescription Handling

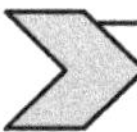 **3.1 Introduction**

A medical prescription is a written order (handwritten or electronic) issued by a qualified health care professional e.g. physician, dentist, veterinarian or registered medical practitioner (RMP) to a pharmacist to compound and/or dispense medicine or device to their patient. This order provides an assistance for the pharmacist to formulate and dispense the medicine to the patient. It also provides instructions for the patient on how to administer medicines. The term "prescription" is derived from the Latin word "*praescriptus*." which is comprised of two words "*prae*, -a prefix" which means "before," and "*scribere*," which means "to write." It denotes that prescription is written before a drug is compounded or administered by the patient. A prescription drug is a pharmaceutical drug used for diagnosis, prevention or treatment of a disease that legally requires a medical prescription to be dispensed.

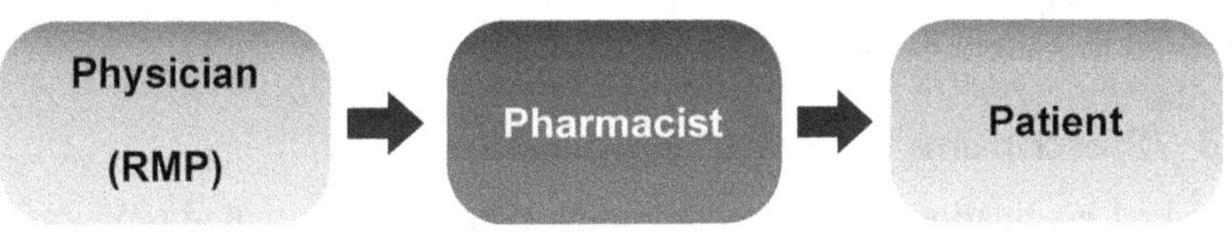

3.1.1 Functions of Prescription

- The prescription can be used as a legal document to purchase the medicine.
- Act as a record for medical history of a patient (cause of illness and its treatment).
- It is required in therapy modality.
- It is a good source of data for clinical trials.
- It is useful to avoid the misuse of the drugs.
- It is used to understand of use of medications in accordance with scientific knowledge.
- It ensures that patient gets right medicine in right does.

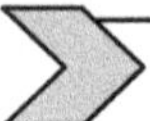

3.2 Types of Prescription

There are three types of prescription:

- Prescription for Extemporaneous preparations (compounded prescription)
- Prescription for Official preparations (non-compounded prescription)
- Prescription for Patent preparations

3.2.1 Prescription for Extemporaneous Preparations (Compounded Prescription)

Compounded prescription are the preparations formulated by the pharmacist in accordance with the order (drug and dosage) directed by the physician. The compounded prescription was followed in the older days which involved the risk of safety of patients. As a result, while preparing and dispensing these medications, practitioners and pharmacists must abide by the Guidelines.

3.2.2 Prescription for Official Preparations (Non-compounding Prescription)

Non-compounding prescription does not require compounding of the pharmaceutical product. The product is available in the market in a ready-to-use form supplied by the pharmaceutical industries and can be directly dispensed to patient by pharmacist.

3.2.3 Prescription for Patent Preparations

Prescribed medications are protected under patent law. Patented preparations are those that are distributed by a firm or company or individual that has a patent on its manufacturing process.

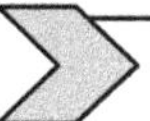 ## 3.3 Parts of Prescription

The prescription is precisely written on a standard format, which is often maintained in the form of pads. The parts of a standard prescription are as follows:

- Prescriber information
- Date of issue
- Patient information (Name, age, sex, and address of the patient)
- Superscription (Symbol R_x)
- Inscription (Main part of prescription)
- Subscription (Direction to pharmacist)
- Signatura or transcription (Direction for patient)
- Renewal instruction
- Prescriber signature and registration number
- Drug enforcement administration (DEA) number

Prescriber information

The information about the prescriber is very important so that he/she can be contacted in case of emergency. Following information must be mentioned on prescription:

- Name of a Doctor
- Address, e-mail, and contact number,
- Any other identifiable details of the prescriber, such as the state licence number

Date of issue

The date has to be written at the top of the prescription which helps a pharmacist to know the prescribing date. It gives a sense of analysis to the pharmacist that when the prescription was written, and the medicine were last dispensed. This avoids the misuse of a medication that is habit-forming or of narcotic nature.

Patient information

The patient information on prescription includes patient's name, age, gender, and address. The patient's name and address are required for the identification purpose and age and gender is used for prescribing the dose. The patient's body surface area (BSA) and weight are also checked in some cases (newborn, a toddler, an older adult, or someone with exceptional needs).

Superscription

It is signified by the symbol R which is written before writing the prescription. The symbol R is an abbreviation obtained from a Latin term *recipere or recipe* which means "Take thou or You take". The symbol was originated in old days from the sign of Jupiter that is considered as Greek god of healing. This sign was used to pray God for the quick recovery of patient.

Inscription

The body of the prescription, or *inscription*, includes the name (generic name or brand name) and strength and amount of the drug to be dispensed. If the prescription has many ingredients, the inscription must be separated into the sections as described below.

a) Base: The active pharmaceutical ingredient(s) (API) having therapeutic benefit.

b) Adjuvant: It is required to enhance the palatability of the product and to increase the action of the medication.

c) Vehicle: It is required to dissolve the ingredients (base and adjuvants) and/or to increase the volume of the formulation.

Note: Now a days, compounding of prescription is not in practice due to availability of medicine prefabricated into dosage forms.

Subscription

It includes instructions to the pharmacist for preparing the prescription. It includes information for compounding, such as dosage form (tablet, capsule, powder), number of doses, packaging instructions, labelling instructions, instructions on allowable refills, and instructions such as "No substitutions" or "No substitutions allowed" when a generic equivalent may not be substituted. All these instructions are nowadays no longer written in the prescription because most of the prescription are not being compounded and dispensed.

Signatura

Oral instructions given to patients are most of the times forgotten. Patient is confused about what dose is to be taken and how often. This consists of direction for the patient (commonly called *Signa* or *Sig* sig) concerning the drug administration. These instructions are printed on the label of the container of prepared formulation. The Signatura includes following instruction:

a) The amount of formulation to be taken (tablet, capsule, syrup etc.)

b) The frequency of administration or application [number of times a drug is to be taken such as, t.i.d. (three times a day), b.i.d. (two times a day), and o.d. (once a day)]

c) The mode of administration (route of administration, and method i.e., one tablespoonful, one teaspoonful etc.)

d) Special instruction (with milk, with water, with an equal quantity etc.)

DEA:................

Name of the Hospital

Doctor's Name
Qualification (M.D.,M.B.B.S.)

Registration No........................
Full Address............................
Contact No...............................
E-mail.....................................

Date:.....................

Name...

age.................... Sex .... Height .... Weight................

Address...

R̥ (Superscription)

Doxycycline capsule................100mg (Inscription)

Dispense 14 tablets (Subscription)

Take the medicine twice a day
Avoid taking with milk   } (Signatura)

Refill: ....

Dispensed by: ....
Date: ....
Name of Pharmacist: ....
Name of Pharmacy: ....
City: ....

**Doctor's Signature
Stamp**

Figure 3.1 An example of a typical prescription

Renewal Instruction

Every prescription should specify if it may be renewed and, if it is, then how many times. It prevents the abuse of prescriptions comprising narcotics and other addictive medications.

Signature and address of prescriber

To confirm the authenticity and misuse of prescription. The prescriber's signature must be on the prescription, with registration number and stamped.

Drug enforcement administration (DEA) number

Number that identifies the prescriber as someone authorized to prescribe controlled substances. (This number is required on all prescriptions for such substances and is often required to file insurance claims).

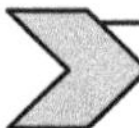

3.4   Legality of Prescriptions

The prescription and supply of drugs of dependence are regulated to minimise harms associated with their use. The misuse of prescription is becoming a critical issue affecting the public health with over 25% of death which is related to opioid drug prescriptions. The verification of prescription with governing rules conforms its distribution. These rules are implemented by the legislation in practice of a particular country which assures the prescriber signature and date on prescription. Therefore, it is the pharmacist's duty to make sure that the signature is authentic and the date is right.

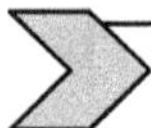

3.5   Prescription Handling

Prescription handling requires a systematic and careful approach to assure that the patient receives the correct medicine in the proper dosage form, dose, and guidance. The pharmacist should examine the prescription thoroughly to verify that it is accurate and clinically acceptable. A standard operating procedure should be followed at all stages of the dispensing process. The following are the steps involved in dispensing a prescription:

- Receiving the prescription
- Clinical and legal checking of the prescription
- Assembly of the product and labelling
- Accurately checking the product against the prescription
- Delivery of the product to the patient with the appropriate advice about the product.

3.5.1   Receiving the Prescription

The patient visits the drug store with the prescription and interact with the pharmacy personnel for medicines. E-prescription is accepted in several countries in this modern age where it is transferred electronically, and the pharmacist gets an electronic document. Upon receiving the prescription, the pharmacist should confirm the identity of the patient, and weather the prescription is presented by patient himself/herself or by someone on the patient's behalf. A pharmacist must not change his or her facial expression after receiving a prescription from a patient because it provides the impression to the patient that he or she is perplexed or shocked after viewing the prescription.

3.5.2   Reading and Legal Checking of Prescription

It is the sole responsibility of the pharmacist to ensure that the prescription is legally complete and clinically correct for the patient. Prescription is reviewed to see which medicines are required and to note patient details. Pharmacy staff should check:

- Patient's name and address
- Age of patient if under 12 years
- Name, dose, and quantity of medicine
- Date
- Prescriber's name and address
- Signature of prescriber
- Legality and authenticity of document

Any missing or confusing information in prescription needs to be checked by the pharmacist before the prescription can proceed to the next stage of the dispensing procedure. The missing information needs to be rectified with doctor either by sending the patient back to the doctor or on phone by contacting the prescriber.

3.5.3   Collecting and Weighing the Materials

In this step, the pharmacist or pharmacy assistant collects the product from the storage sections (selves) and deliver it at the dispensing bench. If the prescription is to be compounded, the material required should be kept on the left side of the weighing balance and then shifted to the right side after weighing. This ensures that all ingredients have been accurately weighed. During this stage, pharmacist intervention to minimize dispensing mistakes includes the following:

- Take caution while picking a medicine; some drugs have nearly identical names. (e.g. – Prednisone and Prednisolone, Amlodipine and Amiloride, Digoxin and Digitoxin, Lescol and Losec).

- Take caution while deciding the right strength of drug; some drugs are available in a different dose (strengths). (e.g. – Paracetamol tablet 325 mg, 500 mg, 650 mg; Atenolol tablet 25 mg, 50 mg, 100 mg, Amoxicillin capsule 250mg, 500mg).
- Take caution while picking appropriate dosage form, a variety of dosage form of a medicines are available (e.g. – Diclofenac tablet, gel, suppositories etc.)

Note: At this stage, errors such as selecting the incorrect strength or form, or even selecting the incorrect product, might occur.

3.5.4 Compounding

The compounding area, as well as any other equipment, should be completely cleaned and dried before proceeding. Only one prescription should be compounded at a time as instructed by the prescriber or according to Pharmacopoeia or formulary techniques. After preparation, the pharmacist should store the preparation in suitable container with an acceptable label.

Note: In the modern method, compounding of prescription is not in practice due to availability of suitable formulations.

3.5.5 Assembling, Labelling, and Packaging

At this stage, labelling of the compounded product is performed by skilled pharmacy technicians. After labelling, the product is arranged in the order they appear on the prescription. The dispenser may be required to keep records at this stage, either for legal reasons, such as completing a controlled drug register, or as a good practice, such as adding data to the patient's medication record.

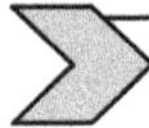

3.6 Labelling of Dispensed Medications (Main Label, Ancillary Label, Pictograms), Brief Instructions on Medication Usage

From the legal perspective, a prescription drug label (i.e., medication container label) comprises of all information provided on the prescription by the RMP. Details to be included on label:

- Patient's name
- Date of dispensing
- Name of pharmacy
- Name of medicine
- Strength
- Dosage form

- Quantity dispensed
- Dose with clear instructions
- Cautionary labels

When many containers of the same drug is to be dispensed, it should be noted on the label that there are multiple containers of the same medicine to avoid confusion. The package insert contains information about the proper use and side effects of the product. Manufacturer provides the information about the product to the pharmacist on the package inserts (comes with all medicines package). These package inserts are legal extensions of the labelling of drug product, and they are subject to the same rules and regulations that apply to misbranding and mislabelling. These inserts are required by FDA regulation to contain the information listed in Figure 3.2.

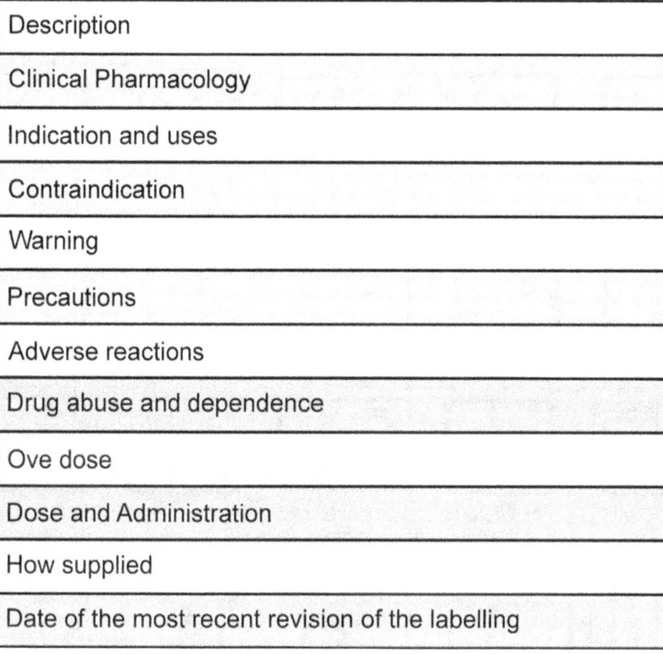

Description
Clinical Pharmacology
Indication and uses
Contraindication
Warning
Precautions
Adverse reactions
Drug abuse and dependence
Ove dose
Dose and Administration
How supplied
Date of the most recent revision of the labelling

Figure 3.2 Organizations of the package insert information

Figure 3.3 Structure of dispensed medicine label

Pictograms

Pictograms are standardized visual graphics that provides medication directions, precautions, and warnings to patients. Pharmaceutical pictograms are graphic signs intended at improving medication comprehension, recall and adherence and reducing the potential risks or errors associated with medication use, particularly in patients with limited health literacy and low level reading ability.

The commonly used pictograms to convey the medical instructions on the prescription are depicted in Figure 3.4.

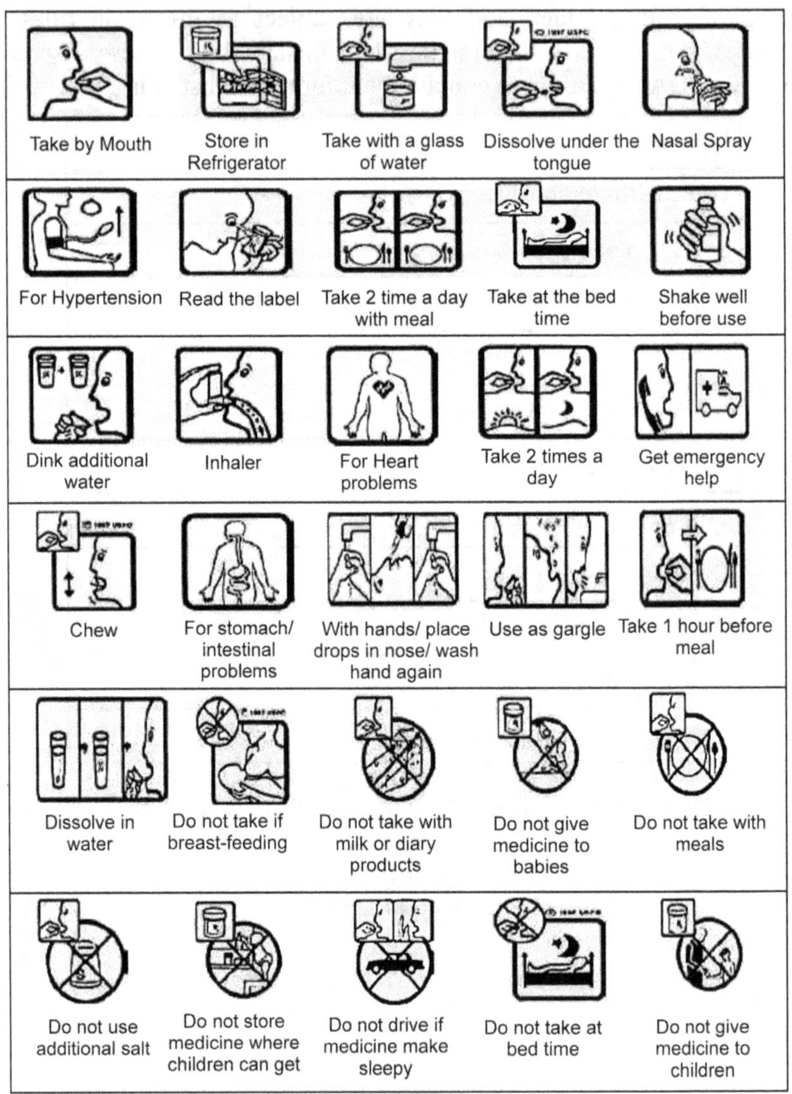

Figure 3.4 Some of the pictograms used while dispensing the medication

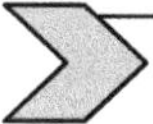

3.7 Dispensing Process

Dispensing describes as the process of preparing and distributing medicines to a designated patient together with instructions, advice, and counselling wherever required. It necessitates the specific clarification of the order for prescribed medicine, its preparation and labelling for the use by patient. The process of dispensing starts while receiving the prescription or request for medicine till it is issued successfully to the patient. While dispensing the medication, the pharmacist must make sure that:

- The prescription is valid according to the specified regulation.
- The identity of the patient is verified and precisely documented in the dispensing software.
- The treatment given should be checked for clinical suitable for patient.
- The information is made available to assure that the drug is used safely and appropriately.
- Pharmacists are responsible for the following during the dispensing process:
- Apply their experience and knowledge, use professional opinion to protect and promote the health, safety, and wellbeing of patients
- Protect the confidentiality and privacy of patients and their related sensitive data.
- In coordination with patients and prescribers, pharmacist improves the clinical outcome.

The process of dispensing involves following steps: (the steps have been discussed earlier):

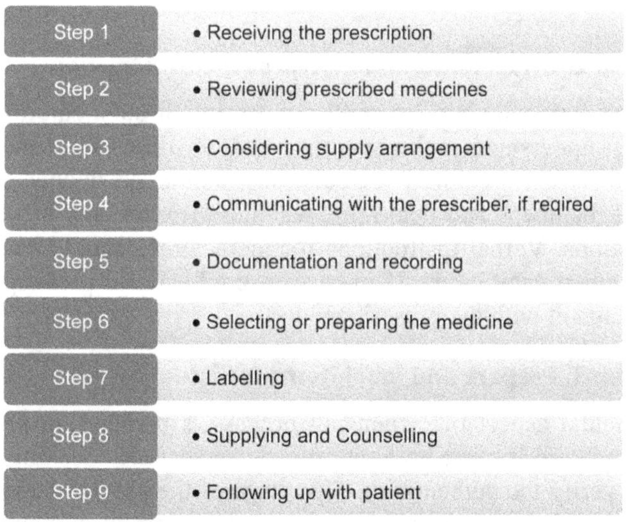

Figure 3.5 Process of dispensing

3.7.1   Good Dispensing Practices

Good dispensing practices ensures that an effective form of precise medicine is delivered to the right patient, in the exact dosage form and quantity, with clear instructions, and in a package that maintains the potency of the medicine.

- Good dispensing procedures must be used consistently and repeatedly to ensure that mistakes are identified and rectified at all stages of the dispensing process.

- The development and implementation of written standard operating procedures (SOPs) for the dispensing process would increase uniformity and quality of work. The six key areas of activity may serve as a basis for such SOPs.

  1. Receive and validate the prescription
  2. Understand and interpret the prescription
  3. Prepare and label items for issue
  4. Make a final check
  5. Record the action taken
  6. Issue medicine to the patient with clear instructions and advice

3.7.1.1   Step 1. Receive and validate the prescription

Upon receiving a prescription, the staff member responsible should confirm the name of the patient. When a prescription is received, the person in charge should double-check the patient's name and identification. It is very necessary to take precaution while dispensing the medicine to a crowd of customers.

3.7.1.2   Step 2. Understand and interpret the prescription

A member of staff who can interpret a prescription must carefully read the prescription, understand abbreviations, ensure dose and dosage form, calculate the dose if required (calculations should be double checked by another staff member), and determine whether there are any prevalent drug-drug interactions. Verbal instructions for medications should be given only in rare and emergency cases. If in-case of confusion in prescription, he or she should consult with the prescriber.

3.7.1.3   Step 3. Prepare and label items for issue

The fundamental aspect of dispensing process is preparation of product(s) for dispensing, and it must involve procedures for self-checking or counter checking to verify the authenticity. This stage of the process begins once the prescription has been thoroughly read and the quantity computed. At this point it will be good to write the label as a form of self-check.

3.7.1.3.1 Select stock container or prepack

During the dispensing procedure, trained staff members read the container label at least twice. A good dispenser chooses the product by reading the label and comparing the product name and strength to the prescription. Holding multiple stock containers open at the same time is another problematic practise that should be avoided.

3.7.1.3.2 Measure or count quantity from stock containers

Liquids must be measured in a clean vessel and poured from the stock bottle while keeping the label facing up instead of down. This prevents any spilt or leaking liquid from damaging the label. Counting tablets and capsules is possible with or without the use of a counting equipment. One of the following methods should be used to count:

- Clean piece of paper and spatula
- Clean tablet-counting device
- Lid of the stock container in use
- Any other clean, dust-free surface

The stock vessel lid must be replaced immediately after measuring or counting, and the stock container label should be cross - checked for medication name and strength.

3.7.1.3.3 Pack and label medicine

A bottle, plastic envelope, cardboard box, or paper envelope should be used to pack tablets or capsules. However, during the rainy season or in a humid environment, cardboard or paper will not preserve pills and capsules from moisture, that can rapidly deteriorate and render them unsafe for use. Capsules and sugar-coated tablets are the most susceptible to moisture.

3.7.1.4 Step 4: Make a final check

The dispensed medication should be verified against the prescription and the stock containers used at this stage. It is preferable to have another staff member for the self-check and final check. Before having a look at the dispensed medications, the final check must include reading and interpreting the prescription; checking the suitability of prescribed doses, drug interactions, identity of the medicine dispensed, the labels; and ultimately countersigning the prescription.

3.7.1.5 Step 5: Record action taken

To run a drugstore properly, documentation of patient are required. Once the prescription is received, the dispenser should record the information in logbook of all the medications dispensed as soon as possible before the products are issued and prescription is returned to the patient. In the record book, the patient's name, age, gender, strength and dose of medicines and name of dispenser must be registered. If the patient uses computer to maintain record, the data must be stored so that it may be retrieved later to compile summary report.

3.7.1.6   Step 6: Issue medicine to the patient with clear instructions and advice

The medication must always be provided to the designated patient, or the patient's representative, along with specific instructions. From patient to patient, the recommended level of informative detail about probable adverse effects varies. Due to the illiteracy and poor labelling issues, the verbal counselling is important. Apart from information on the dose, frequency, route of administration, treatment length, priority should be given to providing information that will maximize the effect of the treatment, it includes:

- When to take the medicine (especially when it comes to food and other medicines)
- How to take the medicine (swallow, chew, take with plenty of water)
- How to store the medicine

Warnings about possible side effects should be given cautiously. Common side effect should be stated to prevent a panicked patient from discontinuing the therapy. More serious side effects should be stated only with the prescriber's permission. It is essential to make every effort to ensure that the patient understands the directions and suggestions. Every patient deserves to be treated with respect. When describing the usage of some medicine, the necessity for confidentiality and privacy must be addressed.

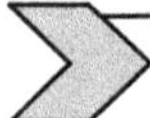

3.8   Sources of Error in Prescription

According to ASHP (American society of hospital pharmacist) guidelines, medication error can be categorized into 11 types.

3.8.1   Prescribing Error

A prescribing error occurs at the time a prescriber commands a drug for a patient. Mistake may include the choice of an incorrect dose, dosage form, route of administration, length of therapy or number of doses. For example: Amoxicillin 250 mg PO TID may be appropriate to treat a middle ear infection in 5-year-old child but would be too high a dose for 12 months old infant and thus would be considered as prescribing error.

3.8.2 Monitoring Errors

Monitoring errors result from insufficient drug therapy review, failure to review a prescribed regimen for appropriateness and detection of problems, or failure to use appropriate clinical or laboratory data for adequate assessment of patient response to prescribed therapy.

3.8.3 Omission Error

Failure to administer a well-ordered dose to a patient in a hospital, nursing home, or other facility before the next scheduled dose is considered as an omission error. Omission is not an error If there is any medical reason When patient cannot take anything by mouth prior to a procedure or Patient refuses to take them.

3.8.4 Improper Dose Error

It occurs when a patient is given a dose that is greater or less than the prescribed dose. Cause of improper dose include delay in documenting a dose or absence of documentation, inaccurate measurement of an oral liquid is also an improper dose error.

Following are excluded from this category are:

a) Doses that cannot be precisely measured

b) Not specified as in topical application.

c) Metric conversions are excluded.

3.8.5 Unauthorized Drug Error

Administration of a medication to a patient without proper authorisation by the prescribers categorised as an unauthorised drug error Causes:

a) If a medication for one patient was given, incorrectly to another patient

b) Nurses give a medication without a physician order

c) Patients at home who sometimes share prescription

d) Refilling a prescription that has no refills remaining without authorisation from the physician

e) Administering medication based on specific patient parameters, by nurses may be wrong

f) Administration of medications outside the established guidelines

3.8.6 Deteriorated Drug Error

Prescribed medication or administered outside their expiration date or may have lost potency or less effective or ineffective. The error may also occur when the refrigerated drugs stored at room temperature, this may decompose where efficacy is less than optimal, so observing expiry date and storage of products are very important

3.8.7 Wrong Time Error

Timing of administration is crucial for the efficiency of medications, maintaining satisfactory blood level of drug is required for effectiveness, administering doses too early or too late may affect the drug serum level and subsequently the efficacy of the drug may affect. Wrong time errors are unavoidable because the patient is away from the care area for a test or the treatment is not available at that time

3.8.8 Wrong Dosage Form Error

Doses administered or dispensed in a different form from that ordered by the prescriber are classified as wrong dosage form errors. The Change in the dosage forms may be acceptable to accommodate patient needs. e.g. - Dispensing a liquid formulation without specific prescription to a patient who has difficulty swallowing tablets might be an acceptable dosage form change.

3.8.9 Wrong Drug Preparation Error

Drugs requiring reconstitution, dilution or special preparation prior to dispensing or administration of drug but fail to do that procedure causes wrong drug preparation error. e.g.- Cephalexin oral suspension with an incorrect volume of water can be considered as wrong drug preparation error.

3.8.10 Wrong Administration Technique Error

Doses that are administered using an inappropriate procedure or incorrect technique are categorized as wrong administration technique errors. Some examples of such errors include, a subcutaneous injection that is given too deep, an IV drug that is allowed to infuse via gravity instead of using an I.V pump.

3.8.11 Compliance Error

Inappropriate patient behaviour regarding adherence to a prescribed medication regimen.

3.8.12 Other Error

The other errors include, calculation error, decimal points error, abbreviation error, and incompatibilities etc.

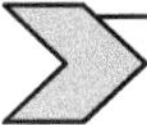 **Exercise Questions**

Multiple Choice Questions

1. The term Rx is an abbreviation of a Latin term which means.......

2. .... is the main part of a prescription that contains the name and quantities of prescribed drugs.

3. Direction for the administration of drugs to patients comes under..............

4. The abbreviation used for water is..............

5. Let a mixture be made in Latin is known as..........

   a. aa   b. ad

   c. aq.   d. ac

6. The Latin word 'cibos' mean

   a. Food   b. with food

   b. After food   d. Before food

7. The abbreviation for h.s. is

   a. Hour   b. Minutes

   c. At bedtime   d. Morning

8. Match the following

   Parts of the prescription   Significance

   a. Signature   1. Name and quantity of the prescription

   b. Superscription   2. Direction to patient

   c. Inscription   3. Avoids misuse of prescription

   d. Date   4. You take

9. Convert the Latin word to English

   a. Charta   b. Dosis

   c. Hora Somni   d. Collunarium

   e. Ter in die   f. Post cibos

   g. Semi hora

10. Convert the English word to Latin

    a. A spray solution

    b. Give

    c. An ointment

    d. When Necessary

    e. When the cough is troublesome

    f. For the eyes

Answers

1. You take
2. Inscription
3. Signature
4. c. aq.
5. Fiat Mistura
6. a. Food
7. c. At bedtime
8. a. 2. , b. 4. , c. 1. , d. 3.
9. a. Powder

   b. A dose

   c. At bedtime

   d. A nasal douche

   e. Thrice a day

   f. after lunch

   g. half an hour
10. a. Nebula

    b. Da

    c. Unguentum

    d. Sis opus sit

    e. Tussiurgente

    f. Oculis

Very Short Answer Type Question

1. Define the term 'Prescription'
2. Define the term superscription.
3. What are the different types of prescription?
4. What is the function of prescription?
5. What do you understand by subscription?
6. What do you understand by transcription?
7. What do you Omission error?
8. What is the purpose of using a Pictogram?
9. Why does the prescription be interpreted by the pharmacist to the patient?
10. Define wrong time error?

Short Answer Type Questions

1. What is the significance of age in the prescription?
2. What is the importance of dispensing medicine in the modern method?
3. Describe the modern method of prescribing a drug.
4. While handling the prescription how does compounding of the prescription takes place?
5. What is the need to refill information in the signature?
6. Explain unauthorized drug error.
7. What is the precaution taken by the pharmacist while dispending the medicine?
8. How does the labelling of medication done?
9. Explain the prescription written for the extemporaneous preparation
10. What is the purpose of the drug enforcement administration (DEA) number?

Long Answer Type Questions

1. Describe the various parts of a prescription and a typical prescription label.
2. Explain the process of prescription handling?
3. How does the labelling of the dispensed medication take place?
4. Explain in detail the modern method of dispensing the medicine?
5. What is the major source of error?

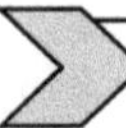 **CHAPTER 4**

Communication Skills

4.1 Introduction

Communication is an essential element of pharmacy practice, both in community pharmacies and in other health care settings. The ability to communicate effectively is vital to providing pharmaceutical care, including identifying patient needs, developing solutions, and ensuring patient agreement. Each individual has a unique way of communicating. A person may use a variety of channels, styles, or ways to communicate information during the communication process. The act of communicating, however, is not solely dependent on the source producing or disseminating information. Additionally, it depends on how the message is conveyed and how the recipient perceives it. At some point, communication starts. Information generation comes first in the process. The next step is to transfer this information or data into a medium for transmission to the target audience. The person who started the contact has to pay close attention to the nature of information throughout this procedure. The success of their conversation will depend on their communication abilities.

Poor communication skill between pharmacist and patient leads to

- Inaccurate patient medication history

- Inappropriate therapeutic decisions

These lead to patient confusion, patient disinterest and patient non-compliance

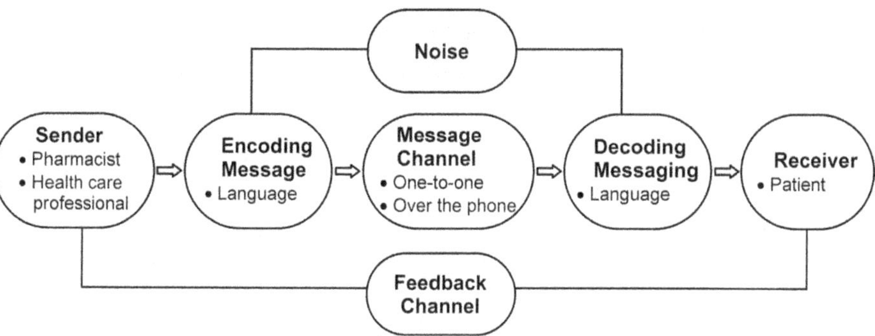

Figure 4.1 Communication Channel

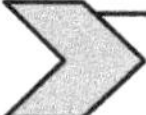 ## 4.2 Types of Communication Skills

While it is easy to think of communication as simply the verbal transmission of information from one person to another, it is so much more than that. While many situations use one singular type of communication, you may find that some communications involve a blend of several different types at once. Communication ranges from non-verbal, such as a glance and raised eyebrows, to verbal, such as a change in pitch and tone. Let's take an in-depth look at all the ways that we communicate with each other.

A. Verbal communication

    a. One-to-one

    b. Over the telephone

B. Written communication

C. Nonverbal communication

    a. Body Language

4.2.1 Verbal Communication Skill

Verbal communication involves language and words to convey the desired message. In general, Verbal communication means communication in the form of verbal language or spoken words only. It is believed that verbal interactions with patients occur the most frequently. Basic verbal communication skills comprise the ability to listen, understand, and respond to what others say as well as the ability to read nonverbal messages and respond in a way that promotes continuing connection. Verbal communication takes place in person or over the phone, and it has the benefit of providing instant response and allowing pharmacy professionals to clarify a statement if necessary. However, in terms of types of communication styles, communication can take either the form of spoken and/or written.

Essential verbal communication skills include the:

- The ability to listen, understand and respond to what others are saying (active listening)
- The ability for interpreting non-verbal cues and reacting in a way that promotes interaction (evaluation).
- Keeping eye contact, nodding, asking questions, etc

One-to-one communication

When one person speaks or writes to another person, it is called one-to-one communication. This occurs when a care provider interacts with a person who is concerned about their health or other issues, such as during a doctor-patient visit. One-to-one communication also happens when healthcare workers interact with one other, as well as with the partners, family members, and friends of those who are getting treatment. One-to-one communication works best when the participants are both at ease and able to switch between talking and listening in turns. Effective communicators are good at:

- Beginning the one-to-one interaction with a friendly, relaxed greeting
- Focusing on the objective of the interaction
- Ending the interaction helpfully and positively.

The communication and interpersonal skills of a practice nurse at a physician's office could be used to know about the symptoms of a patient's health issues, or the patient may have received advice or direction from the nurse on a particular area of their health behaviour or lifestyle. Communication will be more effective if you can establish a positive connection with the service user and treat them with respect while also communicating clearly and in a language they can understand.

Advantages of one-to-one interaction

As there is a tight restriction on confidentiality, one benefit of working one-on-one is that a definite connection of trust may be established. For instance, if the one-to-one conversation is taking place for medical purposes. The conversation is also quite direct, so there is no chance that the individual would feel ignored. Another benefit is that a client may be openly asked questions and express their feelings without fear of being overheard. Individuals typically believe that they can get to know one another better and be more direct to get more information more readily when there are just two other people around.

Over the Telephone

Conversation over the phone is an essential element of oral communication. The emergence of the digital era has sparked a boom of innovation that has given both customers and those who supply healthcare services increased access to a wide range of life-changing medical advancements. There is perhaps no area of the healthcare system that has undergone more significant change than pharmacy and the technology-driven telepharmacy profession. Since most firms have a telephone set on practically every table, it is clear that phone conversations have become a crucial element of communication in the healthcare sector. The delivery of pharmacist care to patients at a distance via telecommunications and information technologies (such as telepharmacy) has shown promise in terms of enhancing patients' access to healthcare services. Telemedicine may be used to provide pharmacist-based patient care services, and it is convenient and cost-effective. Patient adherence to medication for chronic diseases can be improved by personalized telephone counseling from a pharmacist.

Advantages of over the telephone communication:

- An increase in the quality of services and patient satisfaction
- Enhances clinical role for pharmacists
- Expanding pharmacy assistance
- Increases medication adherence
- More widespread use of pharmaceutical services
- Reduces operating costs
- Services provided by a pharmacy with a high level of quality

Disadvantages of over the telephone communication:

- The primary drawback of tele-pharmacy is the lack of total control over how patients are prescribed drugs.
- It is challenging to prevent the use of unauthorized drugs or the distribution of medications without a valid prescription.
- The possibility of violating the regulation of pharmacy practice still exists.

4.2.2 Written Communication

In health care, writing frequently serves as a stimulus for action. Pharmacists are typically recognized and compensated for work that was first initiated by written documents, such as updating patient records, communicating with insurers, and responding to questions regarding medications. Pharmacy professionals may achieve long-term success by maintaining accurate written records, particularly when it comes to compliance and liability concerns. With the advancement of new healthcare technologies, writing is becoming more important. Pharmacists must be proficient writers since most health care communication now takes place on online platforms and in electronic medical records.

Writing annual reports assessments, progress notes, care plans, documents, flyers, treatment guidelines, pharmacy and therapeutics formulary reviews, patient education handouts, flyers, posters, pharmacy legislation reviews, proposals for new clinical services, and drug information reviews. Along with these, pharmacy professionals must be able to write letters to editors in journals, letters of recommendation, articles to be published, or newsletters. A written message should therefore be thoroughly designed to prevent communication gaps and should only be employed for a certain type of receiver when necessary. The stages of written communication include the following:

Stages of written communication

Time management is very crucial during communication because the communication lasts for a few minutes in pharmacy practice. Consequently, good writing contributes directly to positive patient outcomes, the goal of any health care professional. The stages of writing communication include the following:

(i)   Introduction

(ii) Opening

(iii) Business

(iv) Closure

Introduction

It is the first and most important stage to communicate with the patient. Communication at this level tends to repeat itself because pharmacy professionals typically engage with a variety of patients. When communicating with co-workers or medical professionals, the introduction stage will be of the least importance as they may already be acquainted. To have good communication in later phases, the pharmacist should be aware of language barriers and any other expected challenges to communication during the initial conversation.

Opening

It is the second stage. The subject under discussion needs to be introduced and briefly discussed in the second stage.

Business

The main message and information are provided and communicated at the third stage of written communication, and the patient's anticipated data is collected.

Reconnection

The preparation for ending the interaction is part of the fourth stage, which is reconnection. To ensure that the patient or medical professional understands the details and significance of the communication and obtain clarification, the pharmacist will benefit from this.

Closure

The final step is closure. Nonverbal communication is crucial during closure. It provides a hint on when the communication should end. The session will end with a quick handshake, a smile, and a bye gesture.

4.2.3   Non-Verbal Communication

In this type of communication, messages are relayed without the transmission of words. The messages here are wordless. This form of communication mainly aides verbal communication. It supplements it with gestures, body language, symbols, and expressions. Through these, one may communicate one's mood, or opinion or even show a reaction to the messages that are relaying. One's non-verbal actions often set the tone for the dialogue. You can control and guide the communication if you control and guide the non-verbal communication. Some of the modes of non-verbal communication are:

Nonverbal communication happens person-to-person and is as important as verbal communication because technicians interact with patients to a greater extent and attempt to influence their behaviour in roles such as the new medicine service and medicine use. In nonverbal communication, the message is transmitted through our body language, personality, and tone of voice.

The key part of effective nonverbal communication is the capacity to read other people's body language accurately as well as the ability to alter one's body language in response, in effect, to read and convey emotions appropriately during an interaction.

Physical Non-verbal Communication

This is the whole of what can be physically observed. For example, eye contact, touch, gaze, body language, facial expressions, voice tone, posture, and others. Physical nonverbal communication comprises approximately 55% of our everyday conversations. As part of our biological structure, we can detect these small signals. For instance, resting your head on your palms denotes extreme disappointment or rage.

Paralanguage

This is the skill of interpreting hidden meaning. The tone of one's voice is the primary method of such communication. The aim of communication is facilitated by the manner of speaking, voice quality, stress, emotions, or intonation. These features are also nonverbal.

Appearance

Setting the tone is the initial impression. People will respond to the way you look. Your patient's response may influence by your appearance, the colour of your clothing, and other factors.

Nonverbal communication happens person-to-person and is as important as verbal communication because technicians interact with patients to a greater extent and attempt to influence their behaviour in roles such as the new medicine service and medicine use.

Table 4.1 Elements of non-verbal communication

Eye contact	It indicates confidence, attention and honesty
Face expression	An important indicator of emotional state
Body posture	Message can be conveyed through body posture
Tone of voice	Soften voices etc can also influence the communication
Proximity/closeness of position	The pharmacist and patient must maintain a minimum distance of 45cm
Another form of non-verbal message	To convey information through the use of diagrams

4.2.4 Body Language

Body language is a type of communication in which physical behaviours, as opposed to words, are used to express or convey information. Such behaviour includes facial expressions, body posture, gestures, eye movement, touch and the use of space.

The following are some examples of nonverbal (body language) communication.

1. **Eye Contact:** Always maintain eye contact with the patient. However, one must take care to avoid staring at any one individual for longer than five seconds. Eyes that flutter excessively may be a sign of fear. It is not a good idea to stare at someone since it could be threatening.

2. **Crossing your Arms:** Crossing your arms might suggest that a person is not open to discussion, particularly during a patient interview. In contrast, if the interviewer crosses his or her arms during a one-on-one interview, the applicant may do the same.

3. **Sitting Posture:** It is not a good idea to lean on a chair. But one must sit comfortably and straight up. Holding your seat suggests a lack of interest.

4. **Gesture:** A gesture is a kind of nonverbal communication that involves using a body part in conjunction with or without spoken communication. Face expressions, head nodding or shaking, and nodding—which is often seen as a sign of approval, are examples of gestures.

5. **Facial Expression:** The face is the best indicator of a person's emotions. Most of the time, it is simple to tell whether someone is pleased, sad, nervous, annoyed, or enthusiastic. In a professional setting, a person must maintain control over their facial expressions.

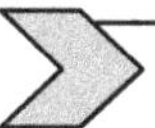

4.3 Communicating with the Health Professionals and Patients

4.3.1 Communication with Medical and Health Professionals

A pharmacist's ability to communicate effectively with other pharmacists, nurses and doctors is important. If the pharmacy practice department at a hospital is newly established, the pharmacist must establish his or her trust in the medical professionals. During communication with health professionals following key points must be remembered:

- Good communication skills and knowledge are the most crucial elements in establishing a better interpersonal relationship.

- Pharmacists should be aware of the doctors' busy schedules and workloads and should avoid unnecessarily detailed information, and focus exclusively on patient-related issues.

- When starting a conversation with doctors about patient care, be ready with specific questions or data and recommendations

- The information provided should meet the standards and clarity. A short and clear statement should provide the necessary information without creating any confusion.

- Pharmacists should avoid any unwanted or irrelevant distractions when collecting information.

- Use nonverbal cues like eye contact, body language, and facial expressions to convey your message.

- Some of the methods utilized for this sort of communication include the telephone and a follow-up document, verbal massage, and written communication in the form of a paper or presentation.

When a patient and a health professional interact professionally, the professionals themselves must likewise act professionally. A health practitioner must be conscious of their reactions in the context of the patient's relationship as well as their knowledge, insight, and awareness of the patient's reactions. A consistent effort must be made to ensure that one's professional behavior is determined by actions that benefit the person seeking assistance in the short and long terms, rather than by one's own needs, and emotions, and desires. This demands a personal approach, empathy, attention, warmth or tenderness, humanism, and respect in the patient interaction. To execute themselves professionally, medical professionals must also be conscious of the patient's dependence on them and the discrepancy in the interactions between them.

4.3.2 Communication with the Patient

Pharmacists are among the most approachable health care providers in the community who provide continual instruction on medication management, monitoring, and guidance to the general public. They must take the patient's requirements and circumstances into account in a professional and ethically responsible manner. Understanding patient views, psychosocial circumstances, and cultural differences are key to patient-centered communication, as is coming to a congruent understanding of patient issues. Miscommunications were also facilitated by a lack of pharmacy professionals, the readiness of practicing pharmacists, and patients' perceptions of practicing pharmacists. To enhance patient health and lower the incidence of medication-related errors, pharmacists should encourage patient-centered communication to build a trusting relationship. However, adherence and satisfaction with the service are influenced by how well patients and pharmacists communicate. Thus, all pharmacists should be capable of transparency, active listening, and simple speaking. Patients must be counseled regarding all aspects of their medication, including the duration of therapy, special instructions and precautions, frequent side effects, therapeutic indications and contraindications, storage and handling, refill details, and the proper course of action to be taken in the case of a missed dose, for both prescription and over-the-counter medications. This will have a favourable effect on patient compliance. Additionally, pharmacist counseling can considerably lower hospitalization and healthcare expenses.

In a professional context, the patient and pharmacist and healthcare provider communicate in a caring relationship. A care relationship is described as a relationship between a human being acting in the role of a patient and a human being acting in the capacity of a professional career. The concept can then be coupled with appropriate traits, such as "caring" or "uncaring," or it can stay neutral. The relationship between the pharmacist and the patient could be described as a complex of attitudes, expectations, and behaviors attached to roles and expressed through interactions. A caring relationship includes the following:

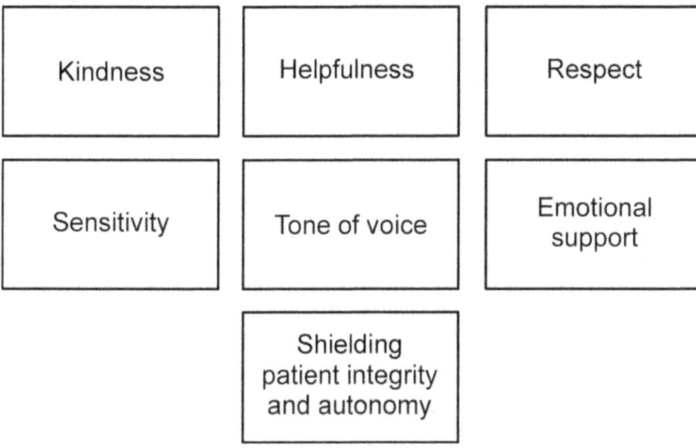

Figure 4.2 Elements of caring relationship

Tips for good counselling by a Pharmacist

- Be relaxed and attentive. Always lean forward while talking to the patients that show their interest.
- Keep the facial expressions relaxed and cool.
- Maintain a balance while standing.
- Move purposefully; it shows confidence. Use hands above the waist. Use both hands and make large gestures.
- Keeping the palms up is a positive gesture.
- Smile when appropriate; look pleasant and genuine, this shows the warmth and openness of the counsellor
- Always turn the face towards the patient facing head vertically up.

Pharmacist Should Avoid

- Gestures like crossing the legs, swinging foot, and tapping fingers reveals that the counsellor is impatient and not interested.
- Avoid shifting eyes and head quickly during a conversation when the patient asks a question.
- Avoid hair twirling, this shows that the counsellor is incompetent and uncertain.
- Don't place the hands in front of the mouth or rub the arm or leg, this shows that the counsellor is in anxiety.

- Avoid talking too loud or too low
- When talking to the patient do not look down or look fiercely the face, this shows that the counselor is defensive and untrustworthy.
- Avoid biting nails, and rubbing eyes and noses.
- Do not look down or to the side. Look directly at the person with a sense of confidence but not threatening in nature.

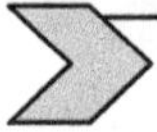

4.4 Patient Interview Techniques

The patient interview serves as the main source of getting detailed information about the patient in terms of providing excellent patient-centered care and the pharmacist's expertise is part of the medication history. A methodical approach is utilized to gather information from the patient, often beginning with identifying the patient's major complaint, sometimes referred to as the reason for the healthcare visit, and then examining the patient's specific complaint and issue. In-depth systemic examinations, potential physical examinations, and questions about the patient's social, personal, familial, medical, and prescription histories are all included in a thorough patient interview.

4.4.1 Medication History Interview

The medication history is the element of the patient interview that gives the pharmacist a platform to use their knowledge by carefully collecting each element of the medication history (A medication history may, however, be obtained without first conducting a thorough patient interview). The pharmacist may find the precise way, time, and reason a patient takes each drug, as well as any adverse reactions, allergies, or problems with medication cost the patient may have encountered, by asking the patient the right questions and using the right method.

The following details are noted during the patient interview:

1. Drugs that have recently or are currently being prescribed.
2. The purchase of OTC drugs.
3. Vaccinations
4. Traditional or alternative treatments
5. A description of adverse drug responses and allergies.
6. Drugs that have shown to be ineffective.

Table 4.2 The five-step model of patient-centered interview

Steps	Description	Actions to improve patient-centered interaction
1	Set the stage for the interview	• Welcome patient, use patient's name, clinician introduction of him/herself • Ensure patient privacy and readiness. • Remove barriers to communication • Assure patient comfort
2	Identify the main complaint and plan the visit's schedule.	• Specify any available time • Obtain the patient's list of issues being discussed. • Summarize the agenda and prioritize the issues for the present meeting versus the future meeting.
3	Open the history of present illness (non-focused)	• Use open-ended questions to bring out issues • Practice active listening, which includes quiet and nonverbal support.
4	Continued the patient-centred history of present illness (focused)	• Use open-ended questions to bring out issues • Practice active listening, which includes quiet and nonverbal support.
5	Transition to the clinician-centred process	• Summarize the discussion and check the accuracy of the data • Explain to the patient that the nature of the inquiry will change from this moment onward (medical questions regarding your symptoms").

Exercise Questions

Multiple Choice Questions

1. When someone is talking and someone else is listening is called……………

2. …………… describes all forms of human communication that are not verbal.

3. Which of the following is NOT a type of communication?
    a. Visual
    b. Mental
    c. Written
    d. Oral

4. Which of the following is an example of written communication?
    a. Tweeting an apology to a customer
    b. A Power Point presentation
    c. A verbal presentation
    d. A letter or memo

5. The effectiveness of communication is usually decided based on
    a. Quality of feedback
    b. Sender's intention and criteria
    c. Economic use of the medium
    d. Simplicity of message

6. Communication problems are otherwise Known as
    a. Enquire
    b. Barriers
    c. Encoding
    d. Decoding

7. The exchange of ideas between two or more Persons is
    a. Understanding
    b. Telling
    c. Communication
    d. Speaking

8. Which of the following is NOT a form of Non-verbal communication
    a. Body language
    b. Tone of voice
    c. Facial expressions
    d. Telepathy

9. The person who transmits the message is called….
    a. Sender
    b. Receiver
    c. Pharmacist
    d. Patient

10. Facial expression are part of
    a. Sign language
    b. Body language
    c. Verbal communication
    d. None of the above

Answers

1. Verbal communication   2. Paralanguage
3. B   4. D
5. A   6. B
7. C   8. D
9. A   10. B

Short Answer Questions

1. What is communication? What are its different types?

2. What are the advantages and disadvantages of over-the-phone communication?

3. Explain about the body language.

4. What is written communication. What are its advantages?

5. List the measures to improve communication effectiveness?

Long Answer Questions

1. Write in detail about the different types of communication.

2. Write in detail about the communication of pharmacist with patients and healthcare professionals.

3. Write a note on patient interview techniques.

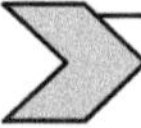

CHAPTER 5

Patient Counselling

5.1 Introduction

Patient Counselling is the practice of giving information, advice, and support to patients so they can utilize their medications properly. The pharmacist provides guidance and information. It is the simplest act to interact with the patient to provide pharmaceutical care. The patient Counselling program is unique because it involves a network of patient counsellor to make sure that both educated and uneducated patients receive good healthcare advice so they may live happy lives. Hospitals select patient counsellor who are qualified to help rural and underprivileged patients who require medical care at every stage of the process. Patient counsellor provide the underprivileged the courage to seek medical attention.

Their roles include:

- The assistance of patients during admission and discharge.

- Counselling patients about the course of their care and providing support during their hospital stay, whether they are inpatients or outpatients.

- Counselling regarding referral services, etc.

Additionally, the patient counsellor provide informational, educational, and communication materials, promote a tobacco-free lifestyle, organize health checkup camps, and perform surveys at the hospital and throughout the community to engage and inspire people to follow pictorial warnings.

5.1.1   Objective of Patient Counselling

- Improve patient understanding of the disease, and side effects of the drug and improve adherence.
- The patient can be encouraged to participate in improved care and self-care.
- Pharmacist should ensure better patient compliance
- Establishing a working relationship and a basis for ongoing communication and consultation
- The patient becomes an educated, effective, and active participant in the management of their health.
- A pharmacist should be considered a specialist who provides pharmaceutical care.
- Avoid drug-related problems such as adverse drug reactions and Drug interactions).

5.1.2   Benefits of Patient Counselling

Effective patients Counselling aims to produce the following results:
- Better patient's understanding of their illness and the role of medication in its treatment.
- Improved medication adherence.
- More effective drug treatment
- Reduced incidence of adverse effects and unnecessary healthcare costs.
- Improved quality of life for the patient
- Better coping strategies to deal with drug related adverse effects.
- The improved professional rapport between the patient and pharmacist.

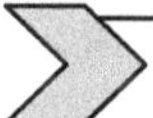

5.2   Stages of Patient Counselling

Counselling is a two-way communication process, and interaction between the patient and pharmacist is essential for Counselling to be effective. The success of Counselling depends on the knowledge and skill of the counselor. Pharmacists should know as much as possible about the patient and his/her treatment details. If the patient is receiving a medication that is unfamiliar to the pharmacist, then a drug information reference should be consulted before Counselling commences. Stages of patient Counselling include the following:

(i)   Introduction (Opening the session),

(ii) Counselling content,

(iii) Counselling process,

(iv) Closing the Counselling session

5.2.1   Step1: Introduction (Opening the Session)

The first step of Counselling is used for gathering information. The pharmacist should introduce him or herself to the patient and greet them by name. Using titles like Ms, Mrs, and Mr. before addressing someone by their first name is the preferred style. The pharmacist should be extremely clear about the session's goal. Pharmacists should know as much as possible about the patient's treatment details. The sources of information in community pharmacies may include the patient, the prescription, or a history of prior dispensing.

A few kind words to express empathy and understanding throughout the Counselling process would help the patient, who may be worried and distressed due to their sickness. If the pharmacist is Counselling a patient, he or she should avoid asking direct or embarrassing questions, demonstrating excessive curiosity, discussing the patient's problems, passing moral judgments, interrupting when they are talking, making premature interpretations, or arguing.

5.2.2   Step 2: Counselling Content

The Counselling content is considered as the key focus of the Counselling session. The pharmacist informs the patient about his or her drugs and treatment plan at this point. Common topics covered include:

- Name and strength of the medication.
- The reason why it has been prescribed, or how it works.
- How to take the medication.
- Expected treatment duration.
- Expected treatment benefits.
- Possible adverse effects.
- Possible medication or dietary interaction.
- Storage recommendation.
- The minimum time frame required to ensure therapeutic efficacy.
- What to do if a dose is missed?
- Special monitoring requirements, for example, blood tests.

5.2.3   Step 3: Counselling Process

The Counselling process is a planned, structured dialogue between a counselor and a patient. It is a cooperative process in which a trained professional helps a person called the patient to identify sources of difficulties or concerns that he or she is experiencing. For the Counselling process, the pharmacist and other healthcare professionals must have good communication skills (Figure 5.1).

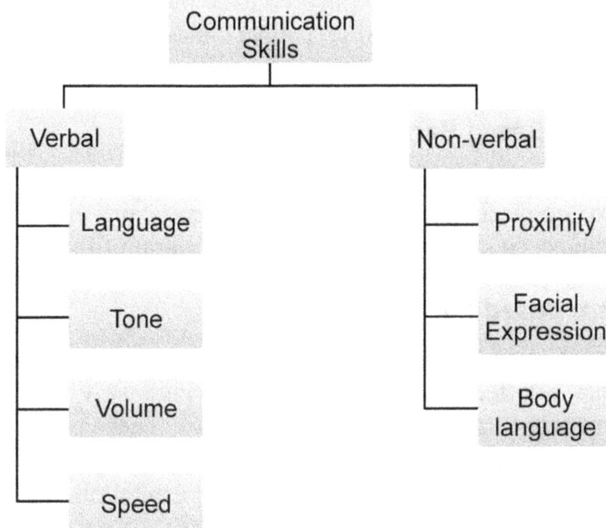

Figure 5.1 Different types of communication skills

5.2.4   Step 4: Closing the Session

Before closing the session, it is essential to check patient understanding. This can be achieved by feedback questions, such as can you remember what this medication is for? Or how long should you take this medication? Ask the patient about any doubts. Before final closure and if time permits, summarize the main point in logical order. Other information may relevantly include previous drug allergies, past medication history, and personal habits such as diet, smoking, alcohol consumption, etc. Use open-ended questions, such as what did your doctor tell you about your illness? what do you know about your disease, can you tell me about the symptoms, etc?

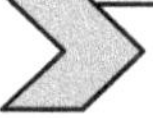 **5.3   Barriers to patient Counselling**

Community pharmacies may not offer patient Counselling due to various barriers. They can be categorized as follows:

- Patient based barriers
- Provider based barriers
- System based barriers

5.3.1 Patient Based Barriers

The vast majority of patients are unaware that pharmacists can offer medication Counselling and generally contact their prescribing physician about medication use. Additionally, patients may be hesitant to ask the pharmacist about medication use due to differences in gender and language.

5.3.2 Provider Based Barriers

Due to a lack of expertise and Counselling skills, many pharmacists lack the confidence to counsel patients. Another significant barrier in many healthcare settings is a high patient load for prescription filling.

5.3.3 System Based Barriers

The majority of places do not have mandated Counselling laws, and pharmacists are not technically allowed to change how medications are administered or what information patients receive. These elements serve as legal and financial hindrances to offer Counselling services. Another issue is the lack of privacy in crowded communities and hospital pharmacies.

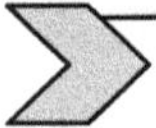 ## 5.4 Strategies to Overcome Barriers

Barriers to patient Counselling can be overcome by using suitable strategies. To practice patient Counselling effectively, it becomes necessary to remove all the barriers that might be felt by the individual. For this, the pharmacist should first identify the barriers and then offer to counsel a patient. Pharmacists should explain to patientswhy they need medication Counselling for better therapeutic outcomes. Overcoming barriers to Counselling requires a good awareness of the wide range of strategies and be open to flexibility in adapting services to meet the needs of their patient.

To overcome the patient based barriers, the following strategies can be implemented.

- Using multi-media materials
- Pictograms
- Oral and written information
- Compliance aids
- Follow up schedules
- Audio-visual tapes
- Tailoring prescription instructions
- Improve communication skills
- Counselling the caregiver through challenges can be learned.
- Overcoming the lack of trust in pharmacists by patient

- Overcoming financial disincentive
- Overcoming privacy and trust issues
- Overcoming gender differences

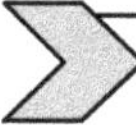

5.5   Patient Counselling Points for Chronic Diseases/Disorders

When specialists provide diagnostic advice to primary care physicians or conduct diagnostic and curative technical interventions without providing ongoing care, they are considered consultants. Preventing drug administration errors is one of the tasks pharmacists can help with in managing chronic diseases. Patients are served by pharmacists by reconciling medications, detecting drug interactions, monitoring drug therapy and prescribed medications, extending prescriptions, and educating them about medications.

When prescriptions are no longer indicated or are no longer beneficial to patients, pharmacists advocate on their behalf. Pharmacists frequently work on nonclinical days to followup with patients who have treatment issues or at the request of nurses and physicians, although they have limited time and financial resources for patient follow-up outside of clinic hours. The participation of pharmacists in the multidisciplinary care team should benefit the patient's recovery in a number of ways, including lowering the cost of prescription drugs for the healthcare system and improving the efficacy of chronic disease management.

5.5.1   Hypertension

Hypertension is a medical condition that occurs when the force of blood flow through the blood vessels is persistently elevated. This makes the heart work harder and increases the pressure of the blood flowing through blood vessels. High blood pressure is a major risk factor for heart disease, stroke, and other serious health problems. Hypertension is generally a disease that develops over years, high blood pressure can be detected early and managed effectively. Hypertension has no initial symptoms, but it can lead to serious health problems, such as stroke, heart failure, and kidney failure.

In order to survive and function properly, tissues and organs need the oxygenated blood that the circulatory system carries throughout the body. When the heart beats, it creates pressure that pushes blood through a network of tube-shaped blood vessels, which include arteries, veins and capillaries. This pressure is the result of two forces:

(i)   The first force is called systolic pressure, and it occurs as blood pumps out of the heart and is carried to the rest of the body.

(ii)   The second force is called diastolic pressure, and it is created as the heart rests between heartbeats.

When your blood pressure is too high for too long, it damages your blood vessels – and LDL (bad) cholesterol begins to accumulate on your artery walls. This increases the workload on your circulatory system and decreases its efficiency. The values for blood pressure measurement are given in Table 5.1.

Table 5.1 Blood Pressure Measurement

Blood Pressure Category	Systolic pressure (mm Hg)	Diastolic pressure (mm Hg)
Optimal blood pressure	Less than 120	Less than 80
Normal	120 - 129	80 - 84
Prehypertension	130-139	85 - 89
Stage 1 hypertension	140 - 159	90 - 99
Stage 2 hypertension	160 - 179	100 - 109
Stage 3 hypertension (Hypertensive crisis)	Higher than 180	Higher than 110

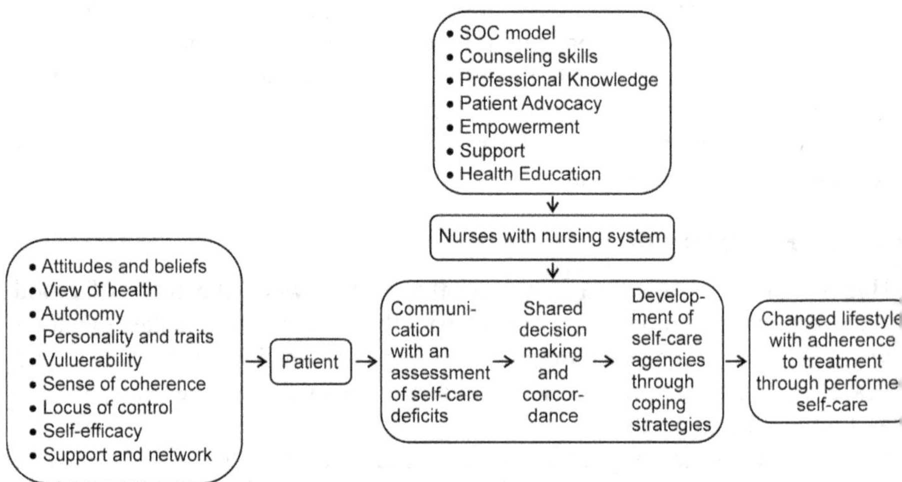

Figure 5.2 The Counselling management model for nurses in hypertension care

5.5.1.1   Counselling Points for Hypertension

Concerning the key points to be covered during Counselling, the following details of Counselling need to be considered:

(i)   **Name, strength, dosage, route of administration:**

Educate the patient briefly about hypertension. Show the patient, the medications prescribed one by one, telling him/her the usefulness of each medication.

(ii) When and how to take medications:

For each medication show and call it by its name; explain to the patient how and when to take medication. Inform the patient's that written directions are fixed to the container of medication. Do not break, crush or chew the tablet. Take the tablet at the same time each day.

(iii) Potential precautions:

Continue taking the drug regularly even if your blood pressure is controlled and normal. Information about adverse effects of each drug needs to be given to the patient (eg. Telmisartan-40 which is usually given as once-daily tablet. The possible adverse effects of Telmisartan-40 include upper respiratory tract infections, sinus infection, back pain, diarrhea etc.).

(iv) Interactions:

Some products that interact with telmisartan, include lithium, ramipril, and drugs that increase the level of K (potassium) in blood like ACE inhibitors, and birth control pills (drospirenone). The patient should inform the physician if he is taking any such medications.

(v) Storage of medications:

Inform the patient about the storage of drugs in a cool dry place away from children.

(vi) About missing dose:

If a dose is missed, the patient may take it as soon as he remembers it but if he remembers it just a few hours before the next dose; then skip the missed dose and take the next dose at a scheduled time.

(vii) Refill information:

Antihypertensives are to be taken regularly without fail. Do not stop taking medicines unless advised by the doctor. Hence, refill information needs to be followed strictly.

(viii) Additional useful information:

Changing lifestyle will also help to reduce blood. pressure such as regular exercise, losing weight, smoking cessation, reducing alcohol intake, and reducing the amount of salt in the diet.

(ix) If the patient has any time questions/concerns encourage him to call/consult a physician.

The management of hypertension requires non-pharmacological as well as pharmacological methods.

Non-pharmacological measures

- In many cases, non-pharmacological therapy by itself may be sufficient to control hypertension.

- A pharmacist can advise to patients on topics such as regular exercise, calorie, and sodium restriction, limiting saturated fat intake while increasing intake of dietary fiber, restricting alcohol consumption, quitting smoking, self-monitoring of blood pressure, and more.

Pharmacological measures

- The majority of individuals need medication treatment.
- Because hypertension seldom manifests any significant symptoms by itself, individuals frequently underestimate it.
- Antihypertensive medications have quite dangerous adverse effects, such as coughing due to ACE inhibitors, bradycardia from beta blockers, etc.
- Drug dose modulation can be extremely important in some circumstances. The pharmacist can use pharmacological interventions such as (Table 5.2):

Table 5.2 Drug Counselling points in hypertension

Drug category	Pharmacist role
Diuretics	▪ Monitor for confusion, dizziness, and muscle weakness. ▪ Make sure the patient is involved in dosage modification. ▪ To prevent frequent urination throughout the night, use the right dosage time. ▪ Describe the potential for ACE inhibitors and drugs to interact.
Beta-blockers	▪ Monitor for hypotension, headache, nausea, and bradycardia. ▪ Inform the patient regarding the potential for nocturnal dreams, impotence, and CNS issues. ▪ Address the necessity of dose tapering before medication discontinuation.
ACE inhibitors	▪ Monitor for hypotension, dizziness, cough, taste disturbances and rash.
Calcium channel blockers	▪ Monitor for chest pain, swollen joints (when taking nifedipine), swollen gums, dizziness, and lightheadedness. ▪ inform the patient to take the extended-release pills all at once. ▪ Inform the patient how to check his heart rate by monitoring his pulse.
Alpha blockers	▪ Monitor for hypotension. ▪ It is important to advise patients using Gastro Intestinal Therapeutic System (GITS) medication not to crush or chew the pills.

5.5.2 Diabetes

Diabetes is a chronic disease that occurs either when the pancreas does not produce enough insulin or when the body cannot effectively use the insulin it produces. Insulin is a hormone that regulates blood sugar. Hyperglycaemia, or raised blood sugar, is a common effect of uncontrolled diabetes and over time leads to serious damage to many of the body's systems, especially the nerves and blood vessels. Gestational diabetes is hyperglycemia with blood glucose values above normal but below those diagnostics of diabetes, occurring during pregnancy. Women with gestational diabetes are at an increased risk of complications during pregnancy and at delivery. They and their children are also at increased risk of type 2 diabetes in the future. Over time, diabetes can damage the heart, blood vessels, eyes, kidneys, and nerves.

- Adults with diabetes have a two- to three-fold increased risk of heart attacks and strokes.

- Combined with reduced blood flow, neuropathy (nerve damage) in the feet increases the chance of foot ulcers, infection, and the eventual need for limb amputation.

- Diabetic retinopathy is an important cause of blindness and occurs because of long-term accumulated damage to the small blood vessels in the retina. 2.6% of global blindness can be attributed to diabetes.

- Diabetes is among the leading causes of kidney failure.

Non-pharmacological approaches

The pharmacist can give an overview of diabetes, stress and psycho-social adjustment, family involvement and social support, nutrition, exercise and activity, monitoring and use of results, relationship between nutrition, exercise, medication, and blood glucose level.

Pharmacological measures

The complications of diabetes can be reduced by tight glycemic control. The drugs used in diabetes are also known to possess certain peculiar features such as being taken half an hour before food in case of sulfonylureas; awareness of hypoglycemia during insulin therapy etc. lists some of the important pharmacological measures a pharmacist should stress while Counselling diabetic patients (Table 5.3).

Table 5.3 Drug Counselling points in Diabetes

Drug category	Role of Pharmacist
Sulfonylureas	<ul><li>Explain the methods to prevent, detect and manage hypoglycemia.</li><li>Monitor for symptoms of jaundice.</li><li>Discuss the administration time concerning food and the need for alcohol abstinence, and ask for a history of sulfur sensitivity.</li></ul>
Insulin	<ul><li>Explain the methods to prevent, detect and manage hypoglycemia.</li><li>Educate the patient regarding newer insulin administration techniques, and proper storage conditions for insulin.</li><li>Ask the patient to carry chocolates or other sweets during travel and ask him not to miss the meals.</li></ul>
Metformin	<ul><li>Advise the patient to take it with/after food.</li><li>Monitor for muscle pain, unusual sleepiness, nausea, stomach pain, and weight loss.</li></ul>
Thiazolidinediones	<ul><li>Take a history of liver problems; monitor the patients for yellow discoloration of urine.</li><li>Monitor the patient for peripheral edema.</li></ul>
Acarbose	<ul><li>Encourage the patient to take it with the first bite of food.</li><li>Monitor for abdominal pain and cramps.</li><li>Advise the patient not to take sucrose (Sugar) during the hypoglycemic attack as it may not be absorbed when acarbose is taken.</li></ul>

5.3.3 Asthma

Asthma is a chronic condition that inflames and narrows the airways in the lungs. The airways are tubes that carry air in and out of your lungs. If you have asthma, the airways can become inflamed and narrowed at times. This makes it harder for air to flow out of your airways when you breathe out.

It affects people of all ages and often starts during childhood. Certain things can set off or worsen asthma symptoms, such as pollen, exercise, viral infections, or cold air. These are called asthma triggers. When symptoms get worse, it is called an asthma attack.

There is no cure for asthma, but treatment and an asthma action plan can help you manage it. The plan may include monitoring, avoiding triggers, and using medicines.

Non-pharmacological measures
- Safety measures while traveling, prophylactic use of drugs before exercise, avoidance of allergens, stopping cigarette smoking, etc.

Pharmacological measures

- Patient involvement in the management of asthma is very important.
- Specific Counselling on drug therapy should concentrate on three areas; drugs to relieve symptoms, drugs used to prevent an asthma attack, and those drugs which are given only as reserve treatment for severe attacks.
- Training regarding the use of the metered dose inhaler is one of the important roles of the Counselling pharmacist.
- The use of these specialized devices is one of the major causes of non-compliance in these patients.
- Many times, the patients fail to take the inhaled steroids, as they do not produce any immediate effects. Some of the pharmacological measures to be included while Counselling these patients are summarized in Table 5.4.

Table 5.4 Drug counselling points in asthma

Drug category	Pharmacist role
Beta receptor agonists	▪ Short-acting drugs belonging to this category should be used mainly for symptom relief. ▪ Patients on long-acting drugs should be told that the medication may take some period to show the action. ▪ Patient also needs monitoring for tremors and muscle pain.
Theophyllines	▪ Patients on sustained release preparations should be told not to crush/chew the tablets.
Anticholinergics	▪ Monitor for dry throat, nausea, headache, blurred vision, and painful urination.
Corticosteroids	▪ Medications should be administered regularly. ▪ They should not be stopped abruptly. ▪ It needs dose tapering before stopping. ▪ Emphasize gargling of mouth after use of inhaled medications.
Mast cell stabilizers	▪ The patient should be told that this medication is used to prevent an asthma attack and it does not relieve bronchospasm that has already started.

5.5.4 Tuberculosis

Tuberculosis (TB) is a bacterial infection that is also known as TB. It can be fatal if not treated. TB most often affects your lungs but can also affect other organs like your brain. Symptoms of TB depend on where in the body the TB bacteria are growing. In cases of pulmonary TB, it may cause symptoms, such as chronic cough, pain in the chest, hemoptysis, weakness or fatigue, weight loss, fever, and night sweats.

The word "tuberculosis" comes from a Latin word for "nodule" or something that sticks out.

The germs are spread through the air and usually infect the lungs but can also infect other parts of the body. Although TB is infectious, it doesn't spread easily. You usually have to spend a lot of time in contact with someone contagious to catch it.

Non-pharmacological measures

- A pharmacist counsel the patient to follow good hygiene practice, use supplement and vitamins, wearing a mask while sneezing and coughing.
- Patients should be made aware of the fact that TB is curable and treatable.
- Once TB is diagnosed, the patient should be screened for other diseases such as diabetes, HIV etc.
- Patients must be informed of likely adverse events during therapy and costs.

Pharmacological measures

- A pharmacist can advise a TB patient on their course of treatment, the best drug regimen for their condition, and any potential drug interactions with their anti-TB medications (Table 5.5).
- Patients should be advised not to stop taking first-line medication therapy despite mild adverse effects that may occur during the first few weeks of therapy.
- Maintain strict surveillance over patient nutrition, infection control, and medication adherence.
- Patients must be advised about how to respond to negative side effects so they know when to consult their doctor and when to stop taking their medications.
- To ensure effectiveness and reduce resistance, pharmacists should adopt Directly Observed Therapy (DOT).
- If necessary, pharmacists should assist in delivering community-level support or mental health services once treatment has started.

Table 5.5 Drug Counselling recommendations for Tuberculosis

Drug Category	Counselling Points
Isoniazid	<ul><li>Tell people to take this medicine on an empty stomach,</li><li>Tell them to take the medication for the full period that has been prescribed.</li><li>Describe any symptoms that might become better as a result of your treatment.</li><li>If a dose is missed, get advice from a doctor since this may make the drug less effective.</li><li>During isoniazid therapy, advise patients to avoid consuming any meals or beverages that have extremely high tyramine or histamine content.</li></ul>
Ethambutol	<ul><li>Instruct the patient to take this medicine at least 4 hours before taking any aluminum-containing antacids.</li><li>Even if your symptoms go away, ask to keep taking this medicine until the entire advised dosage has been used.</li><li>It is advised to take this medicine at regular intervals for the greatest results.</li></ul>
Rifampicin	<ul><li>Instruct the patient to take rifampin at least an hour before taking any antacids if they are taking them.</li><li>Inform the patient that taking hormonal contraceptives while receiving therapy with rifampicin may reduce their efficacy.</li><li>Inform the patient not to combine this medication with praziquantal.</li></ul>
Pyrazinamide	<ul><li>Identify any medications to which the patient may be allergic, including pyrazinamide.</li><li>Find out whether the patient has ever had diabetes, gout, liver, or renal illness.</li><li>Inform people to avoid extended sun exposure or to apply for sunlight protection.</li><li>Inquire about the patient's allergies to other medications, pyrazinamide, niacin, or ethionamide.</li></ul>

5.5.5   Chronic Obstructive Pulmonary Disease (COPD)

COPD is a long-term lung condition that makes it hard for you to breathe. COPD is a common condition that mainly affects middle-aged or older adults who smoke. Many people do not realize they have it. Over time, COPD makes it harder to breathe. You can't reverse lung damage, but lifestyle changes and medication changes can help you manage the symptoms. COPD includes chronic obstructive bronchiolitis with fibrosis and obstruction of small airways, emphysema with enlargement of airspaces and destruction of the lung parenchyma, loss of lung elasticity and closure of small airways.

In developed countries, cigarette smoking is by far the commonest cause of COPD accounting for 95% of cases, but there are several other risk factors, including air pollution (particularly indoor air pollution from burning fuels), poor diet, and occupational exposure.

(a) Non-pharmacological measures:

- The pharmacist should use a disease risk assessment questionnaire to check for COPD in the patient.

- The role of the pharmacist is to counsel patients and educate them about the dose, treatment goals, and the value of adherence.

- Encourage the patient to quit smoking, raise knowledge of risk reduction, and offer guidance on nicotine replacement therapy.

- Demonstrate proper techniques with inhaler use.

- The usage of the inhaler and its proper storage conditions must be shown to the patient, and their education must be ongoing.

- Monitor medication non-adherence in patients and intervene as necessary.

- Give suggestions for changing your lifestyle, regarding food, nutrition, and exercise.

- Inform patients of the importance of good air quality and advise them to refrain from excessive outdoor exercise or to stay indoors when pollution levels are high.

(b) Pharmacological measures:

- For the treatment of COPD, a variety of inhalers are employed, such as bronchodilators, inhaled corticosteroids, and combinations (Table 5.6).

- However, inhalable bronchodilators are most frequently used to treat COPD symptoms.

- A metered-dose inhaler (MDI) usually requires the patient to breathe in slowly and deeply. Most MDIs require priming and shaking before use.

- A dry-powder inhaler (DPI) requires a quick and deep inhalation to pull the powdered medicine into the lungs. DPIs should not be shaken.

- Explain the differences between the various types of inhalers. Bronchodilators relax and open the airways in the lungs.

- Always use the bronchodilator first before using a steroid inhaler. Steroid inhalers decrease swelling in the airways of the lungs. Rinse out the mouth with water and then spit it out after using the steroid inhaler.

Table 5.6 Drug Counselling points in COPD

Drug Category	Counselling points
Levalbuterol	▪ Counselling points prescribed.
	▪ Do the dose and frequency of taking this medication. ▪ If not change the dose unless the doctor instructs to do so.
Corticosteroids	▪ Advice that non-adherence leads to the rapid occurrence of exacerbations, Inform about possible side effects: sore throat, cough, mouth infections. inhaler. ▪ Direct patient to rinse and gargle the mouth with water on using Inform about pneumonia risk with of inhaled steroids.
Roflumilast	▪ long-term use Take this medication at around the same time every day. ▪ Do not use roflumilast to treat sudden attacks of breathing problems. ▪ Enquire for mental health, extreme worry, and unusual mood changes.
Methylxanthines	▪ Instruct not to discontinue taking this medication on initial side effects. ▪ Inform to avoid caffeine-containing beverages with this medication.
Azithromycin	▪ Instruct patient using oral tablets and regular suspension to avoid the use of aluminum or management-containing antacids. ▪ Advise patients to immediately report signs/symptoms of hepatotoxicity or Clostridium difficile-associated diarrhea (severe, watery or bloody diarrhea). ▪ Take medicine on an empty stomach at least 1 hour before, or 2 hours after food.
Ciprofloxacin	▪ Instruct patients to report symptoms of tendonitis or tendon rupture, especially if elderly and/or using concomitant steroids. ▪ Advise patients to use sunscreen, avoid tanning beds, and avoid excessive exposure to sunlight as the drug causes phototoxicity. ▪ Advise patients to avoid caffeine during therapy due to enhanced caffeine effects.
Salbutamol Haw	▪ Advise patients on proper inhalation techniques. ▪ Advise patient to report symptoms of atrial fibrillation, supraventricular tachycardia or hypokalaemia. Warn the patient to report symptoms of paradoxical bronchospasm.
Terbutaline	▪ Contraindicated oral use in the treatment or prevention of preterm labor. ▪ Advise patient to inform healthcare professional if she is pregnant or becomes pregnant while receiving terbutaline treatment. ▪ It may cause palpitations, headache, seizures, tremors, and nervousness.

5.5.6 Acquired Immunodeficiency Syndrome (AIDS)

AIDS is another problem in a health care system already riddled with problems. In the era of widely available anti-retroviral therapy, it is also commonly recognized as a chronic disease that can be successfully managed on a long-term basis. The human immunodeficiency virus (HIV) is the primary cause of the chronic, sometimes life-threatening condition known as AIDS. HIV interferes with your body's capacity to fight disease and infection by weakening your immune system. HIV is a sexually transmitted disease (STI). Additionally, it may be transferred by sharing needles, injecting illicit substances, and coming into touch with contaminated blood. Additionally, it can be passed from mother to kid when she is pregnant, giving birth, or feeding. Without treatment, it can take years for HIV to progressively impair your immune system to the point where you get AIDS. HIV/AIDS has no known cure; however, drugs help manage the infection and stop the disease's development. International organizations are attempting to promote the accessibility of preventative strategies and treatment in resource-poor nations. Antiviral therapies for HIV have decreased AIDS fatalities globally.

(a) Non-medication measures:

- When giving AIDS Counselling, pharmacists should consider the patient's communication style and literacy level.
- Pharmacists should recognize people who may be HIV-positive and promote conversations about ways to cope with knowing one's HIV status.
- Inform people on how to avoid HIV transmission and help individuals who are directly and indirectly impacted by the virus.
- Support the patient by providing Counselling, tracking their progress via treatment, advising on changes in their care, and engaging in academic and professional activities.
- Offer Counselling to individuals, couples, and families to prevent and lessen the psychological morbidity linked to HIV infection and illness.
- Advise the patient to adopt a reliable barrier technique when engaging in sexual activity.

(b) Medication treatments:

Counselling plans are presented in Table 5.7.

Table 5.7 Drug Counselling points for AIDS

Drug Category	Counselling Points
Zidovudine	<ul><li>Inform the patient that this medication controls HIV but does not cure it.</li><li>Ask patients to continue to take this medication even if they feel well.</li><li>Instruct the patient about refilling this medication well in advance.</li><li>Ask patients if they ever had kidney disease.</li><li>Tell to take this medication 2 hours before/after taking clarithromycin.</li><li>Advise patient to report anemia or bone marrow problems during the use of this drug because it may decrease the number of certain cells including WBC and RBC in blood.</li><li>Advise patient to report to the physician for unusual bleeding or bruising, fever, chills, or other symptoms or if there are new or worsening symptoms after starting treatment with zidovudine.</li></ul>
Abacavir	<ul><li>Enquire patients for allergic reactions to this medicine or any of its ingredients in abacavir tablets or solutions.</li><li>Ask the patient aboutthe existence of any chronic disease. Inform interactions of this drug with alcohol, methadone, and orlistat. Advise the patient to continue your normal diet during treatment.</li><li>Advise patient to report signs/symptoms or side effects of this drug to doctor.</li></ul>
Didanosine	<ul><li>Instruct the patient to take this medication on an empty stomach.</li><li>Instruct the patient to shake this oral liquid medication before taking it.</li><li>Take this medication at least 30 minutes before or 2 hours after they eat. Inform the patient to swallow this delayed-release capsule medication and not to break, crush, chew, or open it.</li><li>Advise patient to take this drug on an empty stomach, as the presence of food in the stomach prevents the medicine from being absorbed properly.</li><li>Advice to follow doctor's instructions carefully when taking tablets/capsules of this drug.</li><li>Advise patient not to take didanosine with allopurinol or ribavirin medications.</li></ul>
Emtricitabine	<ul><li>Advise patient to take this medicine once a day with or without food Emtricitabine at around the same time every day. Instruct patients to continue to take emtricitabine even if they feel well.</li><li>Advise patient to avoid co-administration of emtricitabine and lamivudine-containing products.</li></ul>
Tenofovir	<ul><li>Instruct patient not to mix tenofovir oral powder with liquid.</li><li>Advise patient not to discontinue therapy as the virus may become resistant to medications and may be harder to treat.</li><li>Advise patient not to take a double dose to make up for a missed one.</li></ul>

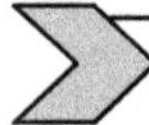

5.6   Patient Package Insert

A package insert is an officially approved document that accompanies a drug and is intended to provide information for its safe and effective use. However, there is a high incidence of medication errors, and the effective use of traditional package inserts is hampered by its complexity and problems of comprehension, for prescribers as well as patients.

5.6.1   Concept of the Package Insert

A package insert is a document, approved by the administrative licensing authority, which is provided with the package of a drug. A package insert, primarily directed at the prescribers, is intended to provide information for the safe and effective use of the respective drug. It is also known as a prescription drug label, prescribing information, etc.

5.6.2   The Patient Package Inserts (PPI)

The distribution of medicines takes place in packages with a predetermined number of units and a fixed strength, a brand name, the responsibility of the holder of the marketing authorization, and an exterior container that inherently connects the package insert to the medication. The patient package insert contains information from a reliable source since the Food and Drug Administration (FDA) has authorized its content following lengthy talks between the pharmaceutical manufacturer, health authorities, and medical professionals from the scientific community.

The PPI is undoubtedly a mass communication tool that is regulated by registration authorities and pharmaceutical companies. However, the patient who receives and reads the insert has been specifically targeted to obtain this particular PPI is essential in cases when verbal means of communication are inadequate. Piece of information by prescription from a doctor and/or delivery from a pharmacist. The specifications for patient package inserts are set by the FDA. Every medication's package insert adheres to a standard structure and contains the same kinds of details. However, various manufacturers may have alternative titles for their sections to make it simpler for the typical person to read and understand, for instance, the part may be entitled "Who should not take this medication?" instead of "Contraindications."

5.6.3   Importance of PPI

PPIs are crucial in enhancing and completing verbal Counselling. It is an efficient way to give people more information about prescription medications. Its widespread use helps to strengthen the pharmacist's position as a counselor. The pharmacist has access to a wealth of patient-related information. They can find out about drugs from a variety of sources, including paid electronic databases, print magazines, and/or free websites.

When looking for medication information, pharmacists frequently struggle to select the best source from the vast number of options. Patient package inserts assist in providing drug information in a conveniently accessible form in such circumstances. As patient package inserts are frequently used by patients for obtaining information about the medicine, the quality and amount of information in them have a significant impact on patient's willingness to comply with their trust. Patient package inserts assist physicians and pharmacists in providing fundamental details on the dosage and frequency of medications, as well as a cautionary note regarding any potential adverse effects. It also provides information on how long the medicine can be kept and how to store the medicine and if not stored properly what it would cause. The majority of information is found in the patient education section of PPI, which has a short and easy form and labeled line drawings. Diagrams, symbols, and images rather than text, such as inserting suppositories or administering eye drops, help poor readers. PPIs that have been carefully formulated are crucial for improving drug understanding, adherence, and therapeutic results. PPIs that are available in regional languages make it easier for regular people to access and comprehend the information.

5.6.4 Benefits of Patient Package Insert

The PPI contains information divided into three sections for patients and healthcare professionals.

- The first section provides information for professionals needed for appropriate prescription and medicine dispensing.
- The second section contains research-related toxicological data as well as data from both human and animal clinical trials.
- The third section includes patient-related information for drug administration.

Other advantages of PPI include:

- PPI assists medical professionals in prescribing drugs appropriately, including educating patients on the drug's uses, contraindications, possible side effects, various forms and dosages, and how to give the medication.
- Information segment in PPIs allows healthcare providers to quickly identify the data needed for patient guidance. PPIs assist patients in properly administering medicine.
- It offers crucial medical information for the usage of OTC drugs.
- PPI information is simple to interpret for educated people.

- PPIs are intended to support or aid patients by using examples.
- The text readability and appropriate arrangement assist the patient in finding the desired information.
- PPI enhances patients' knowledge of medications
- It incorporates more in-depth knowledge about medicines into a perspective of benefits and risks that are balanced.

5.6.5 Scenario of PPI use in India

PPIs are the backbone of approaches for educating people about their medications. PI that comes with drug products in India has to be more standardized and uniform and considered as the primary source of drug information. It is a printed leaflet with information based on regulatory recommendations for the safe and efficient use of a medicine. It is sometimes referred to as the prescription drug label or prescribing information. An effective PI comprises verified, important, and precise details regarding the medication.

In India, a PI is mandated by the Drugs and Cosmetics Rules of 1945 framed under the Drugs and Cosmetics Act of 1940. Sections 6.2 and 6.3 of Schedule D (II) of the Rules specify that the PI must be in English. Although the use of PI is not explicitly stated in the guidelines, it appears to be meant for healthcare practitioners. Pharmaceutical companies in India usually provide PIs for new medications or those that have just been available for around 4 years on the market. However, PIs may still be given for medications that are overpriced (such as biologics and botulinum neurotoxin) or have complex use and administration. However, PIs may still be given for medicines that are costly (such as biologics and botulinum neurotoxin) or have complicated uses and administration (e.g., inhalational or self-administered injectable products). Indian PIs struggle with inadequate information notwithstanding restrictions. The fact that PIs are designed to serve as a protective measure against errors in prescription, dispensing, and administration may be one of the contributing causes to drug errors.

In India, the regularity authority is the Ministry of Health and Family Welfare, Government of India. The complete prescription information is provided by the pharmaceutical companies as part of the marketing application for new drugs application. According to Sections 6.2 and 6.3 of Schedule D, 1940 Act, this information should be provided. After the regularity authorities have accepted the application, the information is incorporated into the package of the medicine. Currently in India, the structure and content of the information on the inserts is geared toward prescribers only.

Given the fact that unauthorized over-the-counter drug dispensing is a prevalent practice in India, and that patient education is in infancy. There is a need for PI to be more patient-friendly and specifically designed to avoid medication errors. India is a country with many languages and most people are not fluent, or even familiar with the English language. User testing of labels and PI is mandatory in many countries, but not in India. Yet, Schedule D about labeling, instructs manufacturers to print labels in English. This point had been taken note of in recent times and the Department of Chemicals of India had instructed manufacturers to print labels in Hindi as well. However, this move met with significant hindrance as Hindi is not a predominant language in many parts of the country. In general, the PI in India needs to improve its structure, content, and language. To enforce the best labeling procedures, regulatory agencies should keep a closer eye on the inserts.

5.6.6 Scenarios of PPI in Other Countries

The idea of a patient package insert has been used in the USA since 1968. This non-technical document included detailed information on the drug, including instructions for usage and an explanation of how it functions. In the United States, this document is also known as "Prescribing Information" or the "Package Insert," and the more informal name for it is "Patient Package Insert."PPI may be necessary for the USA as part of the drug's FDA-approved labeling. To provide clear and simple prescription information, the USFDA, a medication regulating authority in the USA, updated the structure of its package insert in 2006. This latest information is described in Title 21 of the Code of Federal Regulations (CFR), Part 201, sections 201:56 and 201.57, under the heading "Content and Format of Labeling for Human Prescription Drug and Biological Products." All prescription drugs introduced to the market in the USA have to adhere to these rules.

The "Guideline on the Readability of the Label and Package Leaflet of Medical Products for Human Use" was published by the European Commission in 1998. A package insert has been needed for all medications marketed inside the European Union (EU) since 1999. According to European guidelines, patients and the persons who are caring for them should be able to read these information leaflets on their own and/or the contents and directions they get from their doctor or pharmacist. The European guidelines and recommendations govern the content and layout of package inserts to maintain uniformity throughout all EU member states. This makes sure that the dose instructions or potential side effects are mentioned in the same place as the English, Spanish, or German patient information sheet. Articles 59 (3) and 61 (1) call for new requirements for packaging inserts. According to the revised Article 59(3), user consultation is required to show the package insert's readability and use to patients. In the EU, the technical document for drug information is called the Summary of Product Characteristics (SmPQ and the document for the end-user (patient) is the Patient Information Leaflet (PIL) or 'Package Leaflet (PL).

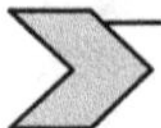 ## 5.7 Patient Information Leaflets

A patient information leaflet (PILs) provides written information about a medicine that is included with every medicine package (Figure 5.2). PILs are sent by the manufacturer by a standard template that contains the same kinds of details for each drug. Their primary objective is to educate patients on how to take their medications, as well as any possible adverse effects and administration instructions.

PILs are typically exhibited at healthcare centers, typically in the waiting rooms, and there is evidence from recent qualitative research that patients value and utilize these health information items. Therefore, a correctly designed PIL has a significant positive influence on patient's adherence to their prescription. PIL is simple to understand for patients because it uses simple language, brief lines, and/or bullet points. Through PIL, pharmacists should ensure that patients are given clear information about risks.

All medications, regardless of how patients obtain them, must have a PIL if not all the information appears on the package. Typically, PIL material consists of the following:

- **Identity of the Medicine:** It discloses the name, the active ingredient(s), the dosage form, and the dose strength of the drug.
- **Therapeutic Indications:** This section outlines the medical problems for which a drug is recommended as well as any benefits that are believed relevant.
- **Prior Information:** This section emphasizes conditions in which the drug should not be used, any precautions, warnings, interactions with other medications or foods, information for certain patient groups (pregnant or, children), and possible effects of the medication on the patient's physical and mental abilities.
- **Dosage:** The information under this section covers how to use or take the medication, the route, and mode of administration, how frequently it should be used, how long the course of treatment will continue, what to do if a dosage is missed, what to do in the case of an overdose, and, if applicable, the risk of withdrawal effects.
- **Description of Side Effects:** It outlines all possible adverse effects that might happen from taking the drug as prescribed as well as what the patient should do if any of them occurs. This information is often given after the order of seriousness and frequency of incidences.

- **Additional Information:** It includes details on the excipients, additional product characteristics, registered pack sizes, storage requirements, and the manufacturer's name and address.

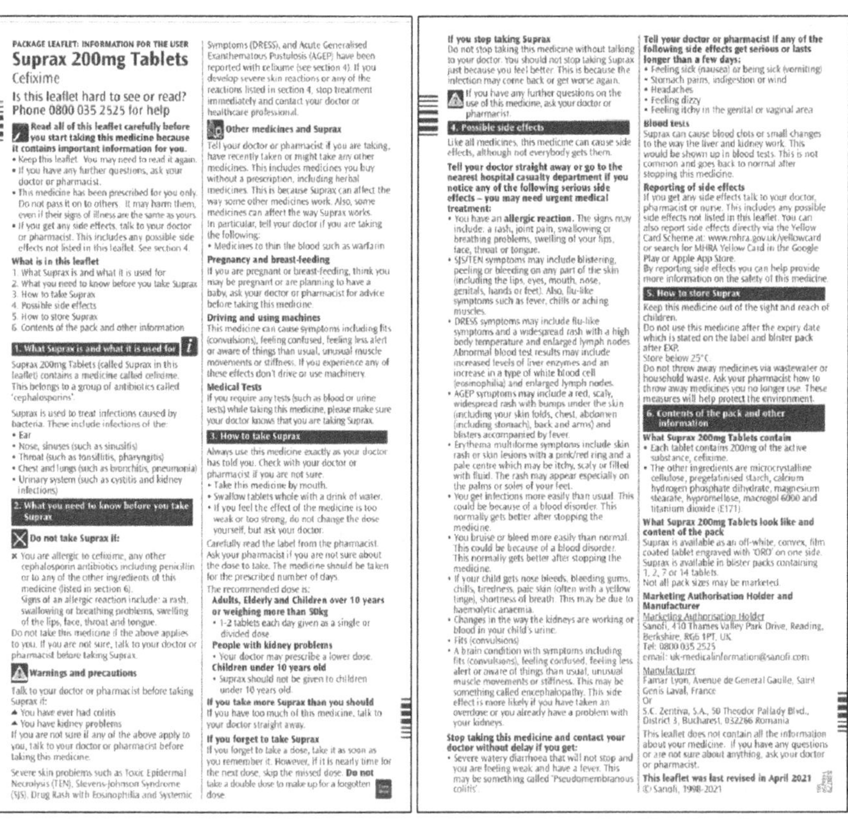

Figure 5.2 Example of PIL

5.7.1   Uses of PILs

From a variety of sources, patients may access a vast range of data regarding health and medications. However, it is frequently difficult for patients to access it. Healthcare professionals often find it difficult to take a break with patients and completely explain what they are going through. PIL gives patients the chance to take charge of their treatment. It is possible to enhance and sustain good health by having an interest in acquiring, understanding, and using PIL knowledge.

PILs can be used for the following purposes:

- By reading PIL, patients can more clearly understand their diagnosis, course of therapy, and/or prognosis and can effectively make healthcare decisions.

- PIL is used to promote patient well-being or to motivate patients to take an active role in controlling chronic diseases.
- PIL provides patients a quick chance to get involved in their treatment.
- PILS are frequently used as reliable sources of medication and health information.
- PILS are used to assist disease prevention, medication therapy, and compliance goals as part of patient education or health promotion.
- PILS assist patients on how to take their prescribed medication, what to avoid, and any possible adverse effects.
- The primary uses of PILS are to promote patient Counselling between pharmacists and patients through communication.

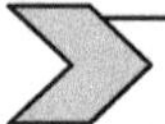 **Exercise Questions**

Multiple Choice Questions

1. When providing patient counseling, what is the primary objective?
    a. To ensure that the patient gets good care.
    b. To meet the patient's needs.
    c. To serve as an intermediary between the patient and their family.
    d. To get non-covered services reimbursed.

2. The _________________ is the heart of the patient counselling session
    a. Preparing for the session.
    b. Opening the session.
    c. Counselling content.
    d. Closing the session.

3. Patient counselling helps to
    a. Know chemical structure of drug
    b. Develop business relations with pharmacist
    c. Motivate the patient to take medicine for improvement of his/her health status.
    d. Pass time at old age

4. Opening of the patient counselling session should include:
    a. Establishing caring relationship with patients
    b. Explain purpose of counseling
    c. Assess the patient's knowledge about his or her health problems and medications
    d. All of these

5. ___________ is a chronic disease that occurs either when the pancreas does not

   a. Hypertension
   b. Diabetes
   c. AIDS
   d. Asthma

6. Theophyllines are given to the patient for the treatment of ....

   a. Asthma
   b. Tuberculosis
   c. Hypertension
   d. Diabetes

7. World Health Organisation recommended a control strategy for TB known as:

   a. DOTS
   b. Gene therapy
   c. Morphine
   d. MCT

8. For Tuberculosis, the drugs used to combat it are

   a. Streptomycin, Pyrazinamide
   b. Isoniazid, Rifampicin
   c. Both (a) and (b)
   d. None of these

9. The main aim of package inserts or leaflets is:

   a. To provide information essential for the safe and effective use of the drugs
   b. Reducing the number of adverse reactions
   c. Adequate direction of use
   d. All of the above

10. COPD stands for ....

11. AIDS is caused by a virus called ....

Answers

1.	b	2.	c
3.	c	4.	d
5.	b	6.	a
7.	a	8.	c
9.	d		

10. Chronic Obstructive Pulmonary Disease

11. Human Immunodeficiency Virus

Short Answer Questions

1. Define patient Counselling. What are its objectives?
2. What do you mean by barriers in patient Counselling?
3. Enlist various components of patient Counselling.
4. What are the methods of patient Counselling?
5. Discuss steps in effective patient Counselling.
6. What are non-pharmacological patient Counselling points for hypertension management?
7. What is diabetes? What causes it?
8. What is AIDS? What causes it?
9. What are benefits of patient package insert?
10. Name factors responsible for COPD.

Long Answer Questions

1. Describe in detail the various stages of patient Counselling.
2. Write in detail about the Indian scenario and international scenario of the patient package insert.
3. Write in brief about the history of PPL.
4. Write in detail about drugs used in the treatment of AIDS. Write patient Counselling points for AIDS.
5. Write in detail about drugs used in the treatment of diabetes. Write patient Counselling points for diabetes.
6. Write in detail about drugs used in the treatment of COPD. Write patient Counselling points for COPD.
7. Write in detail about drugs used in the treatment of hypertension. Write patient Counselling points for hypertension.
8. Write in detail about drugs used in the treatment of TB. Write patient Counselling points for TB.
9. Write in detail about drugs used in the treatment of asthma. Write patient Counselling points for asthma.

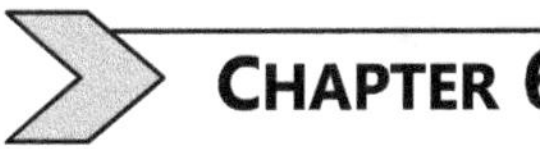

CHAPTER 6

Medication Adherence

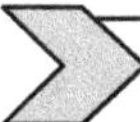

6.1 Introduction

After completing this chapter, students will be able to understand

♦ Analyze patient profiles for medication adherence issues.

♦ Explain reasons for medication nonadherence.

♦ Reflect on pharmacist's value in patient care.

♦ Enhance the role of a patient with a medication adherence issue to foster understanding and patient empathy.

According to the World health organization, medication adherence can be defined as the magnitude of deviation of patient treatment-related behaviour (drug frequency, diet, habits, or refill of drug) from the recommendation given by a medical representative. The term compliance is synonymously used with adherence but differs in meaning. Compliance can be defined as the extent to which the patients follow or obey the instructions given by the health care professionals for the better recovery of the diseases. While adherence is the collaborative work of health care professionals (medical opinion) and patients (lifestyle, values, and preference for care). Many determinants influence drug adherence such as nature and duration of therapy, characteristic of the disease, side-effects of medication, cost, characteristic of health, the severity of disease, facility, and patient perspective about the illness and therapy. Failure to follow such factors leads to non-adherence to the treatment process.

According to National Institute for Health and Care Excellence (NICE) guidelines, non-adherence can be of two types: intentional and unintentional. Intentional non-adherence occurs when a patient deliberately does not follow the treatment recommendation such as omitting a drug, avoiding the prescriber's advice, skipping or altering the dose, etc. while the unintentional non-adherence can be defined as when the patient is unable to take medicine due to uncontrolled barrier such as incompetent to understand prescriber's instruction, inability to pay for treatment, forgets to take medication, etc.

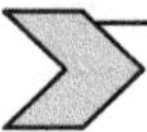

6.2 Factors Influencing Non-adherence

According to WHO the determinants which lead to non-adherence are:

- Socioeconomic (e.g., poor socioeconomic status, illiteracy, unemployment),
- Health system-related (poor medication distribution, inadequate or non-existent reimbursement, or a lack of feedback on performance)
- Therapy-related (complexity of medical regimens, duration of treatments, or the immediacy of beneficial effects)
- Condition related (severity of symptoms, rates of progression, or level of disability)
- Patient-related (knowledge and beliefs, motivations to manage, or confidence).

6.2.1 Socioeconomic Related

When patients have support from their family, and friends to assist with medical regimens, a better adherence can be obtained. Lack of support from family and social networks leads to instability in life that results in less financial resources, difficulty in accessing the medical facility, homelessness, etc. leading to non-adherence.

6.2.2 Health System-related

A good relationship between patient-doctor results in a positive impact on medication adherence. A weak relationship may lead to poor communication, less knowledge of the beneficial effect of the drug, instruction for use, and its side effect. Non-adherence can also occur due to weak memory as in old age.

6.2.3 Condition Related

There is a significant decline in adherence to long-term treatment regimens in chronically ill patients (high blood pressure, osteoporosis, and hyperlipidemia).The main reason for this decline is that there are few or no symptoms. It is crucial that the patient understands the illness and knows what will happen if treatment is not received.

6.2.4 Therapy-related

As a result of the complexity of the medication regimen, which includes taking multiple medications simultaneously and at daily doses; the duration of therapy, lack of immediate benefits of therapy, and interference with lifestyle, treatment adherence has been found to be less than satisfactory.

6.2.5   Patient-related

Nonadherence may be worsened by physical impairments, such as vision, hearing, and cognitive impairments, as well as swallowing problems in elderly patients. Poor medication adherence may be linked to inadequate knowledge about the disease, apprehension about possible adverse side effects, and substance abuse.

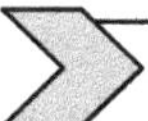

6.3   Strategies to Overcome Non-adherence

Effective treatment depends on the efficacy of medications and adherence to therapeutic routines. Patients with complex treatment protocols and chronic diseases are at a higher risk of not taking the medications needed to adequately treat their ailments. Community pharmacists are in a prime position to have a beneficial impact on patient outcomes and adherence as they are easily available and regarded as trustworthy professionals. Pharmacies may achieve this by advising their customers on how to take their prescriptions.

6.3.1   Educate Patient about What to Expect

In addition to filling in any gaps, pharmacists have the opportunity to provide an extra level of service to patients. The probability that a patient will continue with therapy increases with the number of times pharmacists spend with them discussing the patient's condition, the prescription, and why it's crucial to take it consistently. When patients with chronic diseases believe their medicine is improving their overall health, they are more likely to continue taking it as prescribed.

6.3.2   Nurture the Relationship with Patients

Every patient who enters the pharmacy should be given at least a few minutes of conversation by the pharmacist and pharmacy personnel to build a connection. This action can drastically alter a patient's life. Patients should be asked how they are doing if a new dosage is functioning better, and whether they have noticed any new adverse effects. Such a section helps the patient to stick to their treatment procedure. These dialogs build up trust among the patient.

6.3.3   Team-up with Prescribers

The pharmacy and its customers both benefit from an effective and collaborative workflow. A good healthcare team can more effectively improve the health of patients as a result of the accountable care organization and changing payer supervision that is becoming more common. Additionally, patients will experience the crucial sense of community that comes from being part of a team that routinely discusses their treatment. Many independent pharmacies participate in events outside of their regular business hours, which gives customers the chance to connect with prescribers in person and develop stronger relationships.

6.3.4   Engage the Staff

By frequently having staff meetings and explaining everyone's role in patient care, pharmacists may involve the whole workforce in patient care. Involving the employees and emphasizing the value of managing a patient's care may be done by posting CMS Star Quality Rating3 ratings in the rear of the pharmacy.

6.3.5   Implementation of the Latest Technology

Pharmacies may save a lot of time and money by putting systems in place to monitor and track patient adherence, communicate proactively, and document interactions. The best reporting solutions for pharmacies are those that provide them instant access to patient profiles and historical trend visibility.

6.3.6   Provide a Support Tool

Recognizing the many adherence strategies that are available and how they are positioned to fit a particular patient's preferences can have a noticeable effect on adherence. Some patients could prefer a new smartphone app, while others might think a straightforward daily pill box is perfect.

6.3.7   Patient Compliance

For patients on complicated medication regimens, compliance packaging—grouping all medications into simple-to-manage containers that specify how often and when to take them—might be the best option. Patients are taking charge of their outcomes and looking at solutions for controlling their healthcare in increasing numbers. Make it simple by guiding them, promoting adherence, and maintaining their path.

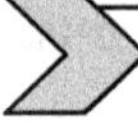

Exercise Questions

Multiple Choice Questions

1. .... is defined as "the extent to which the patient's behavior matches the prescriber's recommendations

2. .... presumes an agreement between prescriber and patient about the prescriber's recommendations.

3. Taking the medication according to the prescription is known as

    a. Medication awareness   b. Medication adherence

    b. Medication avoidance   d. Medication attentiveness

4. Which of the following explain adherence to drug treatment

    a. Filling a prescription

    b. Writing down doctors instruction to consume medicines

    c. Taking the drug as instructed

    d. Knowing the possible side effects

5. Necessary step to be taken when a patient experiences a side effect after following medical adherence

    a. Stop taking drug

    b. Adjust the dose of drug to lower

    c. Report to the medical practitioner

    d. Skip few doses

Answers

    1. Compliance   2. Adherence

    3. b   4. c

    5. c

Short Answer Questions

1. Explain the term adherence and non-adherence

2. What do you understand by compliance?

3. What are the different factors of non-adherence according to WHO?

Long Answer Questions

1. What are the factors influencing medical adherence?

2. Explain the approaches to overcome non-adherence.

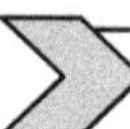

CHAPTER 7

Health Screening Services in Community Pharmacy

7.1 Introduction

As humans, we are concerned about our own health and the health of those we care about on a daily basis. We regard health as our most basic and essential asset, regardless of our age, gender, socioeconomic status, or ethnicity. On the other hand, being ill can prevent us from fulfilling family obligations, working or attending school, or fully engaging in community activities. The level of functional and metabolic efficiency of a living organism is defined as its health.

LEARNING OBJECTIVES

After completing this chapter, students will be able to understand

♦ The term health screening service

♦ Scope and importance of health screening services

♦ Routine monitoring and early detection of disease

♦ Referral of undiagnosed cases

Definitions

a. Health

World Health Organization (WHO), preamble defines health as "a state of complete physical, mental and social well-being and not merely the absence of disease or infirmity". The preamble further states that "the enjoyment of the highest attainable standard of health is one of the fundamental rights of every human being without distinction of race, religion, political belief, economic or social condition".

b. Screening

Screening is the process of looking at a group of mostly asymptomatic people to see if any of them have a high risk of developing a particular disease. Usually, this is done with the help of low-cost diagnostic tests.

c. Monitoring

Monitoring generally refers to the act of observing a disease after a diagnosis in order to assess and improve results, and in certain situations, intervening.

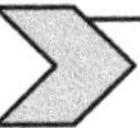

7.2   Health Screening Services and Its Scope

The services that health care professionals offer to check on people's health condition whether or not they have any noticeable symptoms or signs of illness are known as health screening services. To determine the disease or its severity/stage, specific tests are carried out. Nearly all health screening facilities, which are frequently available in community centers, perform these tests. These examinations are commonly referred to as health screening tests. e.g. Estimation of blood glucose, blood cholesterol, blood pressure, lung function test etc.

A doctor may or may not recommend these tests. People can perform these tests by themselves to examine and track their health status because they have no negative effects. In order to monitor health and disease, these tests should carry out on a regular basis. Although not technically a diagnostic tool, health screening tests are frequently used by doctors to decide if you should undergo more focused testing to see if you have a specific illness or are more likely to develop it. In other words, getting screened for diseases shields you from dangers that could otherwise cause issues. Health's screening exam becomes more crucial when:

(i)   a person has a family history of a certain medical condition

(ii)   individual crosses a certain age

(iii)   health risks can be increased by lifestyle

(iv)   a person has a medical history that raises their risk of contracting a particular ailment

7.2.1   Types of Health Screening Services

The health screening tests can be categorized as:

1. Primary health screening

2. Secondary health screening

7.2.1.1   Primary Health Screening

After the commencement of the symptoms, either the patient may undergo these tests on his or her own accord or the doctor prescribes them. These tests aid in the diagnosis of the disease and its severity. Additionally, known as clinical screening or diagnostic screening, primary health screening.

7.2.1.2   Secondary Health Screening

Performed only when doctor recommends such tests. These tests are carried out following the diagnosis of the disease or the disease's stage. These tests are performed to lessen the effects of disease or to monitor its recurrence.

7.2.2 Importance of Health Screening Services

The value of health screenings can be established for a number of reasons because screening tests serve as treatment guides, and the importance of health screening services can be view in terms of following advantages listed below:

7.2.2.1 Identifies Underlying Issue

One of the key benefits of health screening is that it makes it possible to identify when there is an underlying issue, one that has not yet shown symptoms. There may be times when you feel completely well and have not seen any changes, yet there may be a very serious physiologic issue present. Most likely, you haven't noticed it or experienced it yet. Therefore, the value of screening tests depends on their capacity to identify these "invisible" health issues.

7.2.2.2 Helps in Early Detection

The ability of screening tests to recognize some illnesses in their early stages which enables the initiation of treatment for a condition. The chances of a complete and speedy recovery increases with more favorable outcomes. A health check may potentially prolong person's life if they have a serious illness because early detection is crucial in lowering mortality and morbidity rates.

7.2.2.3 Allow Focus on Crucial Area

A screening test clarifies the precise health risks an individual face and informs the doctor to which ones they shouldn't be concerned about. The possible risk regions are reduced, allowing the doctor to concentrate where it is most needed and work without interruption.

7.2.2.4 Catches Sign and Symptoms Before Complications

To avoid emergency circumstances when it comes to health and welfare, the simplest method to accomplish is to schedule routine screening exams as advised by the physician because it catches emerging problems early enough to be resolved before they develop into more serious problems requiring emergency care.

7.2.2.5 Ensures Early Intervention and Less Invasive Treatment

While not always the case, this is generally true for most diseases. Early detection allows the condition to be handled with easier, less invasive treatment options, whether it involves simple health risks like excessive cholesterol or more complicated issues like cancer.

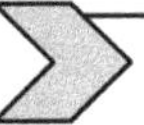

7.3 Health Screening Services in Routine Monitoring of Patients

The routine follow-up and monitoring by medical professionals are beneficial to patients with chronic conditions. Monitoring and follow-up make it possible to regularly assess the efficacy, safety, and adherence of drug therapy and provide ongoing confidence that drugs are assisting patients in achieving their targeted treatment results. It enables the detection of new medication therapy issues. A systematic technique to observe for specific treatment issues is necessary for effective monitoring. Drug therapy monitoring is a continuous process which involves analyzing patient record, identifying and resolving issues arising from drug therapy.

Following routine patient monitoring, a pharmacist may advise the patient to undergo various screenings, such as a routine physical examination, measurements of body mass index, skin checks, blood pressure, eye exams, vaccines, blood glucose testing, and others.

Diseases like diabetes and hypertension requires lifetime treatment. Poor patient compliance, low treatment and control rates, high morbidity, and fatality rates are observed in case of multidrug therapy for treating such conditions. In this instance, regular patient monitoring, raising patient drug awareness, and giving advice on how to take medications will boost patient adherence. The blood pressure and blood glucose levels can be checked by the pharmacist as part of routine monitoring, and they can make the appropriate suggestions, such as contacting a doctor to reduce the dose or change in drug therapy.

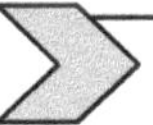

7.4 Health Screening Services in Early Detection of Disease

The likelihood that a disease can be successfully treated or controlled increases with earlier diagnosis. Early diagnosis helps in reducing the number of patient who are diagnosed at late stage. Early detection is essential in order to:

(i) Raising patient's awareness of any initial sign of disease

(ii) Increase the availability and cost-effectiveness of diagnosis and treatment services

Early diagnosis enables the ailment to be managed with simpler, less invasive treatment choices, regardless of whether it includes simple health problems or more complicated issues, thus early detection should be a priority for all individual. Listed below are the benefits of early detection:

(i) It assists in determining who is at danger or has any undiagnosed conditions.

(ii) The likelihood of better health outcomes is increased by early identification, which improves illness management and treatment.

(iii) Age is a significant risk factor for many life-altering illnesses, although early detection can lessen the likelihood of their occurrence.

(iv) Early screening can aid in the prevention of diabetes and cardiovascular disease and can provide access to appropriate treatment if a person has a family history of these conditions.

Examples of some of the health screening tests that are commonly conducted and recommended by the pharmacists for early detection are:

Blood Pressure Test: It is the most important health screening test performed by health care professional for hypertension, while its possible gold standard test is the measurement of intra-arterial pressure.

Cholesterol Test: Recommended for obese and for the individual who frequently consumes alcohol to check their lipid profile.

Diabetes Test: If a person is having a family history of diabetes mellitus, the physician may prescribe tests regarding diabetes for precautionary measures along with the early control of blood glucose level if detected, by undergoing following tests such as blood sugar – Fasting/Post prandial, HbA1c, Glucose Tolerance Test (GTT), insulin resistance test etc.

Mammograms and Pap Smear Test: Mammogram screening is done to examine the breasts, low energy X-rays are used for the purpose of diagnosis and screening for early detection of breast cancer and respectively, pap smear test is done for detecting the cervical cancer in women and the changes in cervical cells that suggest cancer which may develop in future. These tests should be advised to every woman above the age of 60 years.

Colorectal Cancer Test: This test is highly recommended to every individual above the age of 50 years, with changes in bowel habits, stool consistency, abdominal discomfort, blood in stool, colorectal polyps etc.

Prostate Cancer Test: This test is recommended for the individuals having high testosterone levels or those who have obesity. The test should be conducted on individuals age above 50 years for early diagnosis of the condition.

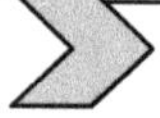 ## 7.5 Referral of Undiagnosed Cases

Being a medical professional, it is the responsibility of a pharmacist to provide pharmaceutical care to the patient and should refer him/her to the other health care provider as and when required, because it is crucial to ensure the patient's continuity of care. Based on patient's medical condition, his health care needs could vary from getting prescription to receiving further treatment. Thus for this purpose, pharmacist after interacting with the patient.

Up-referring is the process of sending a patient to a healthcare professional or facility for care that is more advanced than what is offered in the patient's current setting whereas down referral can be defined as referring a patient to a less specialized facility. In order to stabilize the condition of chronically ill patient, hospitalization or specialized care is required. The patient can be managed and monitored at a facility with less specialized care once the condition has been stabilized and controlled for a while which will reduce the cost of the treatment. The pharmacist should be able to determine those patients who can receive the lower-level care.

When delivering pharmaceutical care, it is important to address the patient's medical requirements holistically, which may involve referring the patient to a social worker, traditional healer, or counsellors for social counselling, this could have an impact on the patient's health and medication therapy.

Patients should be treated as having a medical concern if they are having trouble getting the medications that have been given to them. As part of pharmaceutical care, the pharmacist may identify or analyze the actions and behaviors that calls for referral. The pharmacist is in-charge of informing the institution or other healthcare worker about the referral. The communication, whether it be written or spoken, should include the following:

(i)   A brief synopsis of the patient's medical background

(ii) An overview of the current medical condition

(iii) Details of the referral requirement

(iv) An explanation of the patient's current treatment

(v)   If necessary, a pharmaceutical care plan

To provide pharmaceutical treatment, a pharmacist needs to have a high degree of knowledge and abilities and organizational structure to help with this. In order to give patients better access to pharmaceutical care, the structure must offer referral of patients who cannot be managed at a specific level of care. The pharmacist is responsible for making sure the patient's condition is stable and under control as part of the treatment and care plan. It is necessary to let the patient know where to go and who to visit at the clinic. The health professional and patient should be aware of who the patient is being referred to.

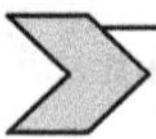 **Exercise Questions**

Multiple Choice Questions

1. The process of looking at a group of mostly asymptomatic people to see if any of them have a high risk of developing a particular disease, is known as

    a. Screening
    b. Monitoring
    c. Controlling
    d. Observing

2. ……………..refers to the act of observing a disease after a diagnosis in order to assess and improve results.

    a. Screening
    b. Monitoring
    c. Controlling
    d. None of the above

3. Health's screening exam becomes more crucial when?

    a. A person has a family history of a certain medical condition
    b. Individual crosses a certain age
    c. Health risks can be increased by lifestyle
    d. All the above

4. The tests when carried out following the diagnosis of the disease or the disease's stage is known as?

    a. Primary screening
    b. Secondary screening
    c. Tertiary screening
    d. All the above

5. Benefits of health screening services are?

    a. Identification of underlying issue
    b. Early detection
    c. Early intervention and less invasive treatment
    d. All the above

6. ……………… test is done for detecting the cervical cancer in women and the changes in cervical cells that suggest cancer

    a. Mammograms
    b. Prostate test
    c. Pap smear
    d. None of the above

7. …………………..is the process of sending a patient to a healthcare professional or facility for care that is more advanced than what is offered in the patient's current setting

    a. Up-referral
    b. Down-referral
    c. Uphill-referral
    d. None of the above

Answers

1. Screening
2. Monitoring
3. All the above
4. Secondary screening
5. All the above
6. Pap smear
7. Up-referral

Short Answer Questions

1. Define the following:

   a. Health

   b. Screening

   c. Monitoring

2. What are health screening services? Write its scope and types.

3. What do you mean by health screening service? What are the advantages of health screening services?

4. Write a descriptive note on health screening service in early detection of disease.

5. What are different health screening tests? What is the need of conducting such tests?

Long Answer Questions

1. Write the scope and advantages of health screening service.

2. Write a detailed explanatory note on health screening services in early detection and routine monitoring of patients.

3. Write a note on referral of undiagnosed cases.

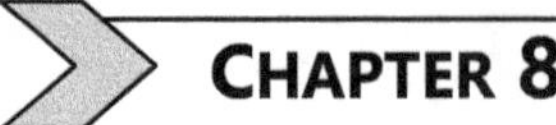

CHAPTER 8

Over The Counter (OTC) Medications

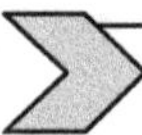

8.1 Introduction

Nowadays patients have developed a mindset of visiting a pharmacist instead of a doctor for minor ailments including common cold and cough, headache, mild fever, acidity, diarrhea, and skin rashes. The purchase of medicine for the above-mentioned condition is recognized as legal in a few countries. Such purchase is referred to as Over the Counter (OTC) medicines which refers to legal permission for the sale and purchase of specific medicine without a prescription. These are also known as Non-prescription drugs which make faster and cheap access to the healthcare service. These are less potent and not dangerous drugs. The only drawback concerns its purchase is its misuse and adverse health effect if consumed in large quantities. For instance, phenylpropanolamine which is found to be present in products used for cold and weight control is abused instead of cocaine.

LEARNING OBJECTIVES

After completing this chapter, students will be able to understand

- Students will be able to learn the definition, need, and role of Pharmacists in OTC medication dispensing

- Students will be able to learn the OTC medications in India, counselling for OTC products

- Students will be able to learn the self-medication and the role of pharmacists in promoting the safe practices during self-medication

- Students will be able to learn the responding to symptoms, minor ailments, and advice for self-care in conditions such as - pain management, Cough, Cold, Diarrhoea, Constipation, Vomiting, Fever, Sore throat, Skin disorders, Oral health (mouth ulcers, dental pain, gum swelling)

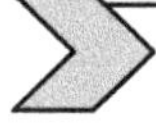

8.2 Need and Role of the Pharmacist in OTC Medication Dispensing

OTC drugs give the general public more affordable access to treatment for minor or self-limiting ailments at a lower cost. The increased awareness among the people have allowed the distribution of OTC drugs for cold, cough, headache, body ache, and itches. In this case, general practitioners (GPs) do not have to write the prescription, instead, patients can directly purchase the OTC medicine from the medical counter. This provides GPs with more time for serious medical problems. This is useful in populated countries like India where the ratio of doctor to patient is very less (1:1800).Though OTC drugs allow faster and cheaper access to the drugs, their misuse and adverse effect are the cause of agonizing. To avoid the misuse of the OTC drugs, the pharmacist can use their professional knowledge to provide a valuable interference in its misuse.

In a country like India where the literacy rate is 74 %, pharmacist plays an important role in forecasting the distribution of the drug among the general public. They help the consumers in selecting the OTC drug for the problem they are suffering. The important role played by a pharmacist are as follows:

a. Pharmacists are the most accessible health care professionals to the patient for the treatment of minor illness

b. They can counsel and provide the appropriate advice on how to consume the OTC drugs.

c. They helps to reduce the burden on general practitioners.

d. They play a vital role in controlling the number of sale on OTC drugs.

e. They help to reduce the drug abuse or overuse of the drug.

f. They also help to avoid any drug interaction which may lead to any adverse reaction.

g. They help to educate and direct the consumers for OTC drugs.

h. They can also advise the patient if found the need for consultancy with the doctor.

i. They can dispense the patient regarding the dispensing practice.

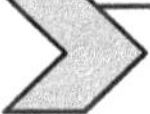

8.3   OTC Medication in India

WHO has defined that for a drug to be sold as OTC it has to be prescribed by the GPs for at least 5 years. This period varies from country to country (New Zealand- 3 years, Japan- 6 years, Philippines – 10 years, and European nation- no specified time). Many countries have differentiated OTC drugs as a separate category with special rules and regulations for their control. It is very important to ensure that the drug is safe to use without causing any side effects during its repositioning from prescribed to OTC drugs.

In India, drugs are regulated according to the schedule reported in the Drug and Cosmetic Act and rule. There is no such regulation for the distribution of OTC drugs, nor any separate category allotted for its sale. The total revenue collected on OTC medication by the Indian pharma market is

1.8 billion in 2009 with an annual growth rate of 10.7%. According to a survey, self-medication of rural population in Maharashtra was found to be 81.5%, Tamil Nadu 23%, Urban Delhi 92.8%, and Odisha 18.72%.

Regulations according to the drug and cosmetics act are as follows:

a. Drugs listed in Schedule H, H1, and X are labeled as drugs to be sold on prescription by GPs.

b. The drugs listed in Schedule G are to be sold under medical supervision.

c. Drugs such as diuretics and aminosalicylate have no distinct division in any category creating a state of confusion among the pharmacist about its sold in the OTC category.

d. Drug present in schedule K includes household remedies such as paracetamol, liquid paraffin, eucalyptus oil, tincture iodine, and formulation for cough and cold which is sold as OTC drugs in India.

e. The nondrug-licensed stores have the authority to sell certain household remedies which fall under schedule K in a village having a population below 1000.

f. The state government of Delhi have declared in 2015 that, Aspirin should be sold only with prescription instead of OTC drugs.

g. The ayurvedic and traditional medicines also fall in the category of OTC, and till now there is no such regulation for their distribution.

Counselling of OTC products by the pharmacist

According to the study in Washington state, counseling the patient regarding OTC drugs has shown a significant result. A pharmacist interacted for 4.6 min on average with 745 patients in a community pharmacy. After counselling, 42.6% of patients changed their intended purchase, 8% cancelled the purchase, 4.3 % decided to consult a doctor and 7.1% learned about the adverse effect (drug-disease interaction, drug-drug interaction, additive side effects, duplication of therapy). Pharmacist counselling helps in the safe and effective use of OTC medication. In order to encourage the pharmacist's work, the American Pharmacists Association society has developed a certificate training program course entitled OTC Advisor: *Advancing Patient Self-Care.*

The counselling to a patient can take place in various modes such as through the driver window, the register, the OTC aisle, the consultation room, or the telephone. The various benefit of patient counselling are as follows:

a. Armed with immense knowledge and a stepwise explanation of self-care, the pharmacist can help a patient to decide on the non-prescribed drugs.

b. The counselling to patients helps them to understand symptoms, characteristics of symptoms, history of symptoms; onset; location; aggravating factors; remitting factors; Medications (prescription, OTC, herbal, dietary supplements); allergies; conditions (medical).

c. It also helps the patient to understand when and how to treat themselves and when to take the physician's help.

d. It helps patients to advise on the appropriate diagnostic tests and when to use emergency health services.

e. It also advises the patient on the proper use of the OTC drugs, with maximum benefit by reducing the risk.

The important steps for counselling a patient include:

a. Effective questioning skills are to be used by the pharmacist for asking a question to patients.

b. The pharmacist should gain as much information from the patient by placing broad, open-ended questions related to the disease.

c. The pharmacist can also place a close-ended question to clarify important points.

d. The pharmacist should avoid asking a question that may lead to false information.

e. The pharmacist should possess active listening skills.

f. The pharmacist should try to gain the trust of the patient by empathizing with the patient.

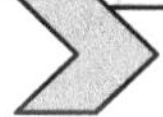 ## 8.4 Self-Medication and the Role of Pharmacists in Promoting Safe Practices During Self-Medication

Self-medication can be defined as the process by which the person takes initiative to intake drugs, herbs, or home remedies by his own will or on the advice of another experienced person. Without any consultation with the doctor. Self-medication can also be understood as a desire and ability of the person/ patient to use his/her intelligence, and independence in decision-making for the management of preventive, diagnostic, and therapeutic activities of any disease. The advertisement in newspapers and magazines act as a source for the self-medication of these drugs. Many governments are increasing the self-medication for minor illnesses. This helps in reducing the cost of treatment, traveling time as well as doctors' time to a major extent. But the major problem associated with this is wastage of resources, increased resistance to pathogens, and serious health hazards related to adverse reaction, overuse, or misuse of the drug. Incorrect diagnosis, misinterpretation, patient confusion, and prolonged suffering. The government should make necessary regulations for efficiently controlling the use of self-medication.

The pharmacist plays an important role in controlling the use of self-medication among the general public. Pharmacists are experts with well-versed knowledge about the action a drug of a drug, its chemistry its formulation, adverse effects, and the way to intake the medicines. The expertise of a pharmacist is well utilized for patient health care. The pharmacist assists the patient with the proper utilization of the medicines and appropriate self-management of the self-limiting and minor conditions. A pharmacist helps in the management of:

a. Management of prescribed drugs: ensuring patient needs to fulfil safety, efficiency, and convenience.

b. Management of chronic condition: provide advice ensuring the patient takes the medicine properly.

c. Promoting a healthy lifestyle: giving advice on healthy living and providing educational materials.

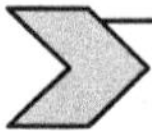

8.5 Responding to Symptoms, Minor Ailments, and Advice for Self-care in Conditions such as

The major role of the pharmacist is to analyse the symptoms carefully of the patient and advise accordingly. The general public has utilized this service provided by highly knowledgeable professionals. According, to the national health service in 1948, medical treatment and its service have become free of cost for the public which reduced the number of public approaching pharmacists for advice. The issue with this was general practioner were spending much of their time with patients having minor issues instead of dealing with complicated cases. To overcome this issue the government introduced the concept of OTC drugs so that they could be purchased in the medical shop without a prescription. The Royal Pharmaceutical Society of Great Britain (RPSGB) officially underlined the role of the pharmacist in the treatment of minor illnesses. With this, the response of pharmacist to symptoms have become important. Many factors make it challenging for responding to symptoms:

a. No access to the patient medical history

b. Have to respond only to the physician's examination.

c. Diagnostic results are not available.

d. A detailed conversation is not possible

e. Privacy issues may be a concern

f. Sometimes symptoms are presented on behalf of another person.

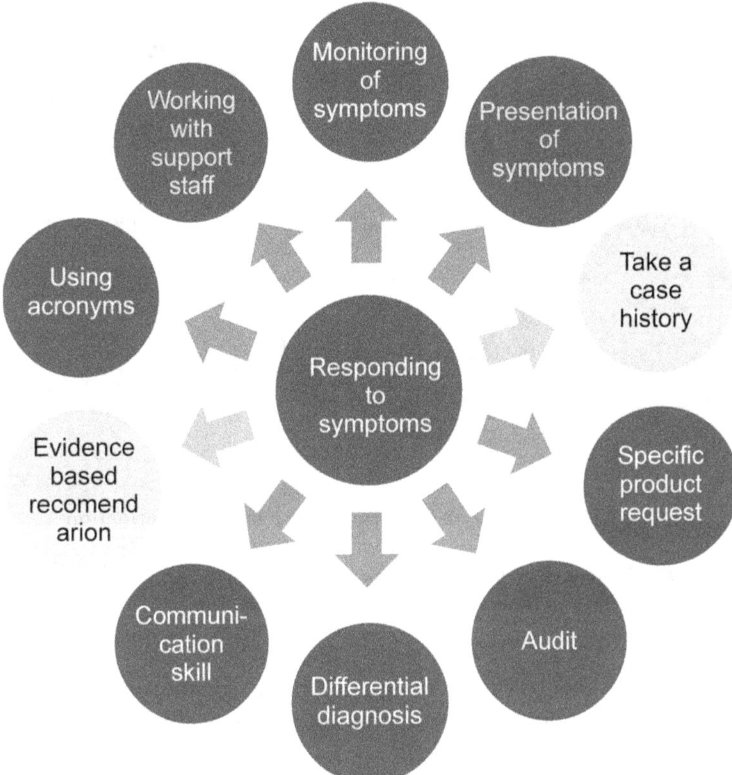

Figure 8.1 Factors to be considered while responding to symptoms

8.5.1   Stages of Pharmacist Response

1. The pharmacist responds in a four-stage manner while dealing with the patient:

   a. Patient assessment: This is based on the information provided by the patient based on the doctor's diagnosis.

   b. Questioning: This process helps to eliminate the more serious condition.

   c. Confirmation: This process helps the pharmacist to confirm the provisional diagnosis.

   d. Recommendation: Suggesting the non-drug or OTC measures or advising proper medical personnel if required in a serious condition.

2. The acronym can also be used to gather information from the patient. An example of an acronym is as follows.

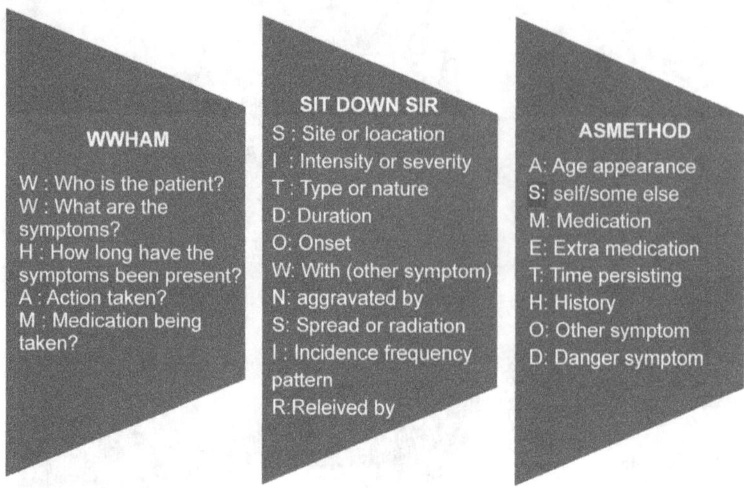

Figure 8.2 The acronym used to gather patients' information

8.5.2 Minor Ailments, Conditions, and Advice to Self-care

8.5.2.1 Pain Management

Pain is a complex and common complaint found in all age groups people. Pain is multidimensional, affecting people physically, psychologically, socially, and spiritually. Self-care is often the first choice for the management of pain. Self-care involves multidisciplinary approaches for treating pain without the involvement of professional health care.

8.5.2.2 Cough and Cold

This is a condition when the body responds to irritation of the throat. An irritant stimulus is sent to the brain, where after processing brain sends signals to the chest and abdomen to expel the irritant out of the lungs. Three basis OTC drugs are available for the treatment of cough: expectorant, suppressant, and combination cough product. The precaution to be taken while using the OTC drugs for cough is:

a. Medicines are not to be taken for more than 7 days.

b. The correct dose should be taken.

c. Drug interaction in the case of combination therapy should be checked.

8.5.2.3 Diarrhoea

Diarrhoea can be defined as loose, watery, and more frequent bowel movements resulting in nausea, vomiting, abdominal pain, and weight loss. If a person does not recover in 24 hr, the body becomes dehydrated, and fever and bloody stool occur in extreme cases.

Keeping the body hydrated by taking water, broth, and fruit juices help to recover from diarrhoea. The doctors recommend sports drinks to maintain the electrolyte balance in the body. There are two types of OTC medications that can be taken in case of diarrhoea: (i). Loperamide (Imodium) helps to slow down the movement of the bowl which helps to absorb water and nutrient from the intestine. (ii) Bismuth subsalicylate helps to maintain the balance of fluid movement out of the body.

8.5.2.4 Constipation

Constipation is the condition in which the bowel movement becomes less frequent and its passage out of the body becomes difficult. These results are due to inadequate intake of fibers or changes in diet. During constipation, the colon absorbs more water from the waste material resulting in solid matter. This situation is common among old age people, women, on medication, or a person suffering from neurological problems. The different health condition that leads to constipation is an endocrine problem, colorectal cancer, irritable bowel movement, neurological disorder, lazy bowel syndrome, intestinal obstruction, structural defect in the digestive tract, and pregnancy. Doctors' recommendation is needed on severe pain, bloody stool, and if it lasts for more than one week.

Recommendation

- It is recommended to take 2-3 extra glasses of water a day.
- Avoid caffeine drinks or alcohol that dehydrates the body.
- Eat more prunes or bran cereal and a fibrous diet like Metamucil, Citrucel, and Benefiber.
- Do more exercise.
- A squatting position in the toilet may help for proper bowel movement.
- Laxative or stool softer recommended by the doctors should be taken.

8.5.2.5 Nausea and Vomiting

Nausea and vomiting are not a disease but a symptom that may arise due to stomach infection, or food poisoning. Motion sickness, overeating, blocked intestine, brain injury, appendicitis, heart attack, and migraine. Vomiting can be defined as voluntary or involuntary emptying of the content of the stomach. Pregnant women or people undergoing cancer treatment are more prone to vomiting. Vomiting is also caused in case of motion sickness, sea sickness, and other kinds of sickness. Excessive vomiting may lead to dehydration, dry lips and mouth, sunken eyes, and rapid pulse rate. Nausea is a condition that creates a sensation of vomiting and discourages one to eat anything. If the vomiting results in black or bloody vomit, severe belly pain, lasting more than 24 hr., inability to urinate, yellowish color of the skin, and high fever, refer to doctor for medical help. OTC medication Bismuth subsalicylate helps to treat nausea and vomiting.

There is a certain precaution that one should take while feeling vomiting and nausea:

- Drink ice-cold water
- Eat light food
- Avoid fried food
- Eat slowly
- Avoid excessive exercise
- Avoid brushing your teeth
- Avoid taking solid food. Stick to a liquid diet
- Proper rest
- Avoid taking oral medicine

8.5.2.6 Fever

Fever is the condition in which the body temperature rises more than normal, usually to 97-99 F (100 F is higher). The temperature of the body is controlled by a part of the brain named hypothallus, which increases the temperature in response to infection, illness, or any other cause. Some of the symptoms related to fever are chilling, sweating, headache, feeling weak, loss of appetite, dehydration, etc. The irregular body condition which results in fever is a blood clot, vaccination, heat exhaust, cancer, and infection in the ear lungs, skin, throat, bladder, etc. A Doctors recommendation is required to identify the cause of the raised temperature. It can be treated at home by taking OTC medication acetaminophen 650 mg suspension twice a day for children/adolescents/ infants. A few measurements which help in recovery are:

- Take plenty of rest and sleep.
- Drinking lots of water so that the toxins are washed out of the body.
- Avoid alcohol as it can make a person dehydrated.
- Wear a light weight comfortable clothes with light bed covers.
- Take lukewarm water.

8.5.2.7 Sore Throat

A sore throat can be defined as pain, scratchiness, or irritation in the throat with the difficulty in swallowing. It can be the result of viral infection such as the common cold or flu. Streptococcal infection is caused by bacterial infection and is a rare type of sore throat. The common sign and symptoms of sore throat are pain or scratchy sensation on the throat, swelling in the salivary gland, difficulty in swallowing, a horse or muffed voice, etc. A doctor's recommendation is needed if a person experiences difficulty in breathing, unusual drooling which results in difficulty in swallowing, swelling in the neck and face, blood in saliva, joint pain, etc. various OTC drugs can be used to treat sore throats. The pharmacist can help to recommend the right medicine. The various measurable steps which can be taken at home are:

- Avoid closeness with the person who has any cold or flu symptoms.

- Maintain cleanliness and wash your hand before eating anything.

- Alcohol-based sanitizer can be used frequently to kill the microbes in the hands.

- Avoid handling public objects such as phones, toilets, doorknobs, light switches, drinking fountains, etc.

- Cough or sneeze into tissue with nose covered.

- Gargle in every 2 hr. with warm water with a pinch of salt in it.

Thus, we can conclude that OTC medicines should be recognized by law and patient awareness programs to support pharmacists and pharmacist companies should be conducted. This will create knowledge about its usage and labeling among the people

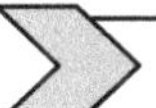

References

- Over-the-counter medicines: Global perspective and Indian scenario

- Patient Counselling: A Pharmacist in Every OTC Aisle

- The role of pharmacy in health care

- Pain Management Guideline

- Basics of Pain Assessment and Management

- Introduction to Community Pharmacy Practice and Responding to Symptoms

- Community pharmacy professionals' practice in responding to minor symptoms experienced by pregnant women in Ethiopia: results from sequential mixed methods

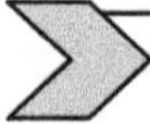 **Exercise Questions**

Multiple Choice Questions

1. What does OTC stand for:
   a. Other tablet and capsule
   b. Occasional therapeutic care
   c. Over the counter drugs
   d. Optional therapies and care

2. The dosage directions on an OTC label are:
   a. Recommendation or suggestion only, not exact instruction
   b. Precise instructions that should be followed exactly
   c. Based on people of average weight and height
   d. All the above

3. How are prescription medicines different from OTC ones?
   a. They contain much smaller amounts of active ingredients
   b. They don't contain dyes or preservatives
   c. They're unsafe for use without medical supervision
   d. They can be toxic

4. You should follow certain precautions when you self-treat with OTCs. What should you do?
   a. Know what symptoms you're trying to treat
   b. Read the label carefully and follow dosage instructions
   c. Follow any label warnings
   d. All of the above

5. If pregnant, the most important part of the OTC drugs facts label:
   a. Warning
   b. Direction
   c. Uses
   d. Inactive Ingredients

Answers

1. c   2. b

3. c   4. d

5. a

Short Answer Questions

1. What is the status of OTC medicine in India?

2. What is the role of pharmacist is promising the self-medication by the patient?

3. What are the different factors to be considered while responding to the symptoms?

4. What do you understand by acronym?

5. Give details of the OTC medication taken in case of sore throats.

Long Answer Questions

1. What are the major ailments, condition and advice to self-care? Explain any three in detail.

2. What does pharmacist counsel a patient about OTC drug?

3. What are the need and role of OTC medication in India?

CHAPTER 9

Community Pharmacy Management

Community pharmacy management is a unique field that focuses on a structured intervention process to study the relationship between the community, pharmacist, patient, and general practitioner. For this intervention, a randomized controlled trial is designed whose primary objective is to manage human resources, finances, marketing, store inventory, information systems, and physical space of the pharmacy. The skill required by the pharmacist to implement this intervention is to manage the interpersonal relationship as well as should possess the strategic foresight to detect changes in the environment.

LEARNING OBJECTIVES

After completing this chapter, students will be able to understand

♦ Students will be able to learn about the Legal Requirements to Set up a Community Pharmacy.

♦ Students will get the knowledge about the pharmacy design and its interior.

♦ Students will be able to learn about the inventory management

♦ Students will also be able to learn customer relation management, SOP of pharmacy management.

♦ Introduction to digital health, mhealth and online pharmacies

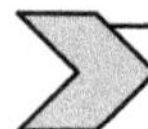

9.1 Legal Requirements to Set up a Community Pharmacy

The sale of the drug is a specified job different from the sale of common goods. This takes place according to Drug and Cosmetic Act 1940 and rules 1945, generating the necessity to issue a license for the sale of medicine. For this purpose, the state government appoints a LA, who has the power to issue a license and grant power to a person under his control. The person who is applying for the license should hold a bachelor's degree or a doctorate in pharmacy from a well-reputed college in pharmacy. For the retail sale of the drug two types of licenses are issued: (i). General license, (ii). Restricted license.

9.1.1 General License

The general license is issued to a person who has the land to do a business and is a qualified person who can supervise the sale of drugs by compounding and dispensing. The drugs specified in schedules C, C_1, and X are issued under form 20, and drugs specified in C and C_1, excluding X are issued under form 21.

The condition associated with a general license are:

- The license should be displayed openly in front of the public.
- The license should be issued according to the Drug and cosmetic rule.
- Any change in the list of qualified staff should be in the knowledge of the authority.
- Precaution for the storage of schedule C and C_1 drugs should be strictly followed.
- Any change in the constitution of the licensing firm should be solely informed to the LA within three months.
- Drugs should be purchased from a licensed dealer and manufacturer.

9.1.2 Restricted License

The drugs that fall under the category of restricted license are those other than specified in schedules C, C_1, and X, and also those specified in C and C_1 but not included in X are issued in forms 20 A and 21 A respectively. The restricted license is issued to dealers, itinerant vendor, or a vendor who purchases drug from licensed dealer.

Condition for restricted license:

- An adequate premised should be selected for the proper storage of drugs to which the license is applied.
- The license should be displayed openly in front of the public.
- The license should be issued according to the Drug and cosmetic rule.
- Drugs should be purchased from a licensed dealer and manufacturer.
- The drugs cannot be sold without the presence of a qualified person.
- Drugs should be sold in their original container.

9.1.3 Site Selection Requirement

The important step in the selection of a community pharmacy is the selection of an appropriate site. A good site depends on the availability of the general public in the surrounding area which adds to its success rate. Important steps to be considered while selecting the site for the community pharmacy are:

- Population ratio of the surrounding area.

- Income distribution of the people living there.
- The flow of traffic.
- Type of pharmacy
- Competition in the area
- Transport facility for raw material, labor, and product
- Electricity and safe drinking water facility
- It should meet all state and federal laws related to the practice of pharmacy

9.1.4 Pharmacy Design and its Interior

The layout and design of a pharmacy are very important. Layout refers to the arrangement of things in their proper specified space and design refers to the color and visual effect given to the pharmacy store.

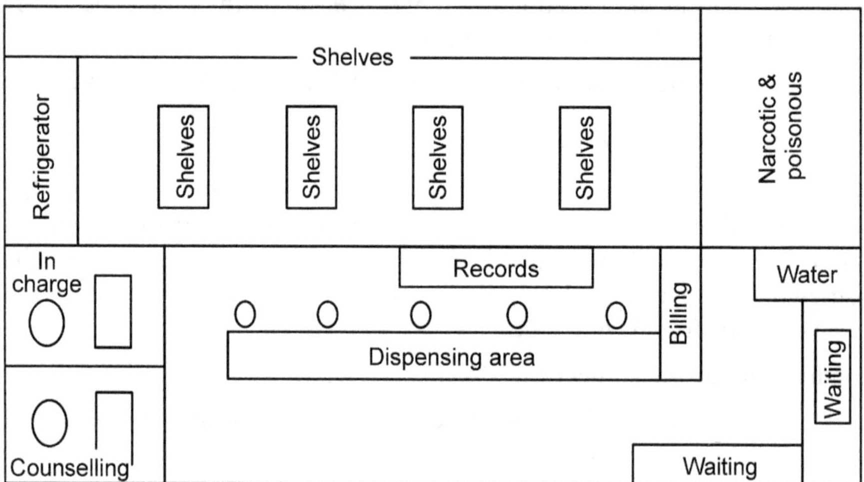

Figure 9.1 Layout of the Pharmacy store

- The floor space should be sufficient for the client to comfortably stand at the dispensing counter.
- Displays and counters positioned in straight, parallel lines will maximize the use of space for selling.
- Modular cabinetry combined with custom casework should be present to store the medicine at room temperature.
- A space should be provided for patient information display.
- A separate area for patient counselling should be provided with a proper chair and table where a patient can freely discuss their doubts with a pharmacist.

- A small area should be denoted for reference resources such as books internet access, etc.
- Additional space should be provided for making extemporaneous preparation with the necessary equipment.
- A well-furnished cabinet should be kept to maintain the patient medication records.
- A well-maintained refrigerator should be present in the pharmacy to store medicines having cold storage.
- Increase the lighting level in the prescription reading area to reduce the mistake in analysing the medicines.

9.1.5 Vendor Selection and Ordering

The vendor's service is a critical aspect of the successful outcome of a clinical study. A pharmacist must specify certain criteria such as cost, delivery of the product, service, flexibility with the consumer, inspection of vendor facilities, availability of returned-goods policies, and availability of institution-specific services. etc for selection of vendor. Prior to receiving the goods or any service for the study vendor's quality management should be checked thoroughly. Before proceeding with any final agreement vendor should know the capacity, identity, capability, stability, experience, etc of the vendor.

9.1.6 Procurement, Inventory Control Methods, and Inventory Management

9.1.6.1 Procurement

The procurement and supply management of goods and services is one of the key factors which is involved in the profit and loss of any organization. A small reduction in the cost of any goods impacts the huge margin of the company. Procurement is a process of identifying and profitably purchasing goods and services by any organization. It is a strategic process that involves identifying needs and requirements, sourcing and evaluating the supplier, purchasing, and covering all the activity till the delivery of goods by the supplier. It also involves the work and services from a third-party vendor in a profitable manner through direct purchase, competitive bidding, tendering process, etc. This process helps to:

- Ensures the continuous flow of raw material at its lowest cost.
- Increase the quality of finished goods
- Satisfy the customer's needs.

9.1.6.2   Inventory Control

Inventory can be defined as the list of materials, quantities, parts, supplies, expensive tools, and in-process or finished products recorded on the stock book by an organization and kept in a warehouse or plant for some time. In other words, it can be explained as a stock of raw material, semi-finished and finished goods maintained by an organization.

Characteristics of inventory

- A business may experience fluctuation in demand or supply of goods which may disturb the working of an organization. An inventory helps to maintain stability in the organization.

- Inventory requires a proper space and also consumes valuable taxation and insurance. Therefore, it is necessary to take care of the stored valuables and sell them at the right time.

- Various decisions such as marketing production, finance, and purchasing decision are directly linked to inventory policies.

- The inventory provides production economics.

Inventory control

Inventory control or stock control is the process to check the stock of warehouse inventory which regulates and maximizes the company's profit. There are many steps involved in verifying inventory and its management such as forecasting, within an organization to meet the demands placed upon that business, including supply chain management, production control, financial flexibility, and customer satisfaction. This helps to produce the right quantity and quality of goods, made available to the users, at the right time, for given production activity, maintenance, or repairs with the minimum of investment.

The objective of inventory control

- Better use of man, machine, and material
- Protection against fluctuation and demand
- Protection against fluctuation in output
- For production economies
- Control of stock volume
- Control of stock distribution

Methods of inventory control

The main purpose of inventory control is to maintain the balance between the cost which increases or decreases with the size of inventory. There are some methods to control the inventory:

- ABC analysis: In this method, the material is classified into three major categories: Group A, Group B, and Group C. Group A consists of highly consumed goods which may be 10 to 20 percent of total items but account for about 50 percent of the total value of the stores. Group B consists of medium consumption items that constitute 20 to 30 percent of the inventory where a reasonable degree of control is needed. Group C consists of very consumed items that constitute 70 to 80 percent of the inventory it costs about 20 percent of the total value.

- Economic Order Quantity: It helps to decide how much inventory should be ordered.

- Just in time: In this method, the inventory is ordered at the time of its replenishment stage. This can create out of a stock situation

- The material requirement planning method: In his method, the inventory is ordered based on previous order sales and demand in the market.

- Vital essential and desirable analysis: Vital items can be explained as those items without which the function of an organization is badly affected. Desirable items are necessary but do not cause any loss in their absence.

Inventory management

Inventory management can be defined as the constant flow of material into and out of an existing inventory. This helps in preventing the inventory from becoming too high or dwindling to levels that could put the operation of the company functioning. This also helps to control the cost associated with the inventory goods included+ tax burden).

9.1.7 Financial Planning and Management

Planning is a comprehensive process that entails carrying out any work or making any decision in a purposeful manner. Financial planning is the phrase used when referring to planning from a financial perspective. It can be defined technically as the process of assessing the required capital and figuring out its composition. It is the process of establishing financial guidelines for the acquisition, management, and investment of an organization's financial resources.

A holistic financial plan takes into account not only your investments and wealth-building efforts, but also your debt and tax obligations, regular spending, family planning, home setup, retirement savings, and the protection of you and your loved ones through appropriate insurance policies and estate planning. Financial planning is a crucial life skill that will enable you to better control your financial goals by assisting you in setting realistic goals, analyzing your options, and taking appropriate action. A prudent plan helps to:

- Meet current financial needs by keeping an eye on your spending and savings.
- Meet your long-term financial objectives by assisting you in charting your life course like owning a house or marriage.
- Having the appropriate insurance plan that will safeguard you and your family in case something goes wrong.
- Build a retirement plan by accumulating sufficient wealth to cover your future expenses.
- Save money by building a retirement nest egg to handle unforeseen catastrophes.

Characteristics of a sound financial plan

- The plan should be simple covering equity shares and simply fixed interest debentures.
- A long-term view is seen while estimating the capital and fund for the organization.
- The financial plan should be adjustable and revised without any difficulty.
- A reasonable amount should be needed to raise the plan.
- Adequate liquidity must be ensured.

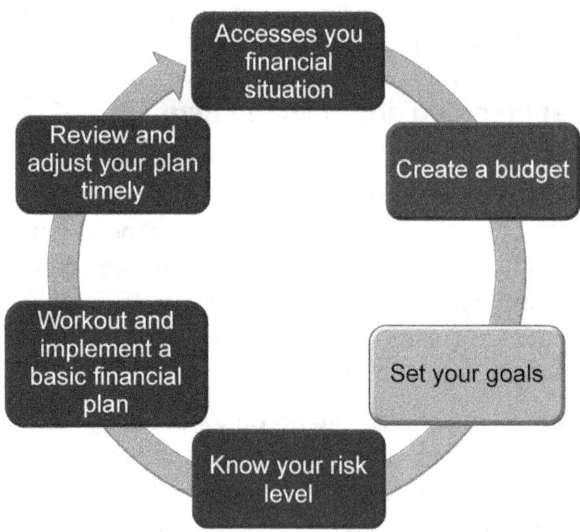

Figure 9.2 Key measure to draw a basic financial plan

Financial management

Planning, organizing, directing, and regulating financial activities, such as the acquisition and use of an organization's assets, are all part of financial management. The purchase, allocation, and control of financial resources are often part of financial management. It entails comprehending the company's financial issues and looking for inexpensive financing options and profitable business ventures. Many methods have been designed to help financial managers suggest the best courses of action. These tools assist the manager in identifying the funding sources with the lowest cost of capital and the ventures that will yield the highest rate of return on investment. There are two methods to assess the objectives that financial management must complete. One classification scheme associates the tasks with the complementary objectives of liquidity and profitability. The second technique of classification focuses on the types of managed assets and funds.

9.1.8 Accountancy in Community Pharmacy – Day Book, Cash Book

9.1.8.1 Day Book

A daybook is a book of original entries where transactions are recorded by date as they transpire in an account. Later, this data is placed into a ledger, where it is compiled into a set of financial statements.

Sales Return Day Book				Sheet no. 34
Date	Customer	Ledger Follo	Credit note no.	Amount

9.1.8.2 Cash Book

An original entry book in which all cash receipt and payment is recorded is known as cash book. The book entry starts in the beginning of the new financial year and is entered timely. There is no cash balance at the start of the session. Keeping a separate book for cash transactions is required since there are typically many transactions involving cash because the majority of business dealings end up being cash transactions. When a cash book is kept, monetary transactions are not recorded in the journal and there is no need to have a cash or bank account in the ledger because the cash book serves as the cash account. Cash is act as both book of original entry as well as ledger.

Types of cash book

- **Simple cash book:** This particular cash book keeps track of all cash receipts and payments. All money received will be reordered on the debit side and paid for on the credit side, whether it be in the form of coin, notes, checks, postal orders, bank draughts, or treasury notes.

Receipts
Payments

Date	Particulars	R.N.	L.F.	Amount	Date	Particulars	V.N.	L.F.	Amount

- **Cash book with Discount columns**: When the cash book has a column for discounts in addition to a column for cash on each side. They are referred to as two-column cash books. The column for discounts shows cash discounts granted to clients on the debit side and cash discounts received from creditors on the credit side. Cash book with bank and Discount columns.

Two column Cash Book

Date	Particulars	R.N.	L.F.	Discount	Amount	Date	Particulars	V.N.	L.F.	Discount	Amount

- **Cash book with bank and discount columns**. Cheques are used to make and receive a lot of payments as the banking industry develops. To keep track of bank accounts in such a situation, the cash book should feature a bank column in addition to the cash and discount columns. The three column cash book can be described as:

Three Column Cash book

Date	Particulars	V.N.	L.F.	Discount	Amount	Bank	Date	Particulars	V.N.	L.F.	Discount	Amount	Bank

9.1.9 Introduction to Pharmacy Operation Software – Usefulness and Availability

The ongoing pandemic have increased the rate of contactless access to the drug. In this situation, pharmacy software is a boon since it makes it easier for pharmacists to operate their businesses. Additionally, it improves the consistency of sales and profit margins. It becomes necessary to ensure that the technology being used is suitable, effective, and environmentally friendly for the benefit of the healthcare system. The huge amount of data produced by pharmaceutical management operations is initially synthesized by the pharmacy operation software. The data is then processed to provide information for usage in organizing tasks, calculating demand, deciding where to put resources and monitoring and assessing pharmaceutical management activities. Following are the benefits of using the pharmacy operation software:

a. **Patient's Medical History:** Retail pharmacy software systems allow pharmacists to keep an eye on patient treatment to ensure they are being dispensed safely. The medical histories of patients are likewise accessible to and reviewable by pharmacists.

b. **Maintain Separate Registers/Folders:** With the use of the pharmacy register system, the pharmacist can keep track of all the drugs maintained in the store. This is an excellent tool because it maintains a record of the drugs and offers alternatives for those that aren't for sale. In an emergency, this is a life-saving alternative.

c. **Identify expired items:** The online pharmacy software system is an excellent approach for identifying expired drugs, as it does not produce bills for expired drugs. This program assists in methodically making new purchases by warning the counter employees about expired medications.

d. **Systematic sales:** When invoicing is done for many batches of the same product, the expiration dates of the products are presented. Based on the FIFO (First In, First Out) and LIFO (Last In, First Out) policies, the appropriate batch of the item is selected.

e. **Barcode labels:** All goods are given a barcode label before being sent to pharmacies and retail outlets. The newest pharmacy software helps to automatically label medications and print expiration dates for drugs. The software also assists in determining the required quantity of labels.

f. **Influence Customer Shopping Behaviour:** All customer information is stored in the pharmacy software's customer relationship management section. The pharmaceutical tool allows proprietors to notify clients via emails and SMS regarding commercial deals and marketing initiatives. By doing this, the owner gains a customer's trust and grows his or her clientele.

g. **Automatic Delivery:** An intriguing aspect of the pharmaceutical distribution software is its ability to automatically distribute orders to different distribution channels based on the goods' supply dates and the number of days required to deliver the order to the consumers.

9.1.10 Customer Relation Management (CRM)

Customer relation management (CRM) is a process in which an organization utilizes a combination of practices, strategies, and technologies to manage and analyze customer behaviour throughout the interaction. It adds value for both the firm and its customers through the appropriate use of technology, data, and customer knowledge. This strategy requires focus, training, and investment in new technology and software to aid in the development of value-adding CRM systems. This helps in attracting new customers, retaining the old ones, and satisfying their needs. This helps to strengthen their relationship with customers and drives sales growth.CRM thereby combines organizational capabilities, people, and technology to provide connectivity between the business, its clients, and partner companies.

Importance of CRM

1. A CRM system includes historical views and analyses of all existing and potential clients. This facilitates fewer searches, customer correlation, effective customer foresight of demands, and growth of a business.

2. Because CRM has all of a customer's information, it is relatively simple to hunt them down and may be used to identify which customers are likely to be profitable.

3. In the CRM system, clients are divided into distinct groups based on their line of work or physical location and assigned to various customer managers, also known as account managers. This aids in concentrating and focusing on every single customer separately.

4. A CRM system is helpful in attracting new clients as well as managing relationships with current ones.

5. Customer Relationship Management's cost-effectiveness is one of its key features. The benefit of a properly executed CRM system is that there is much less need for paperwork and physical labor, which means that there is less staff management and resource management required.

6. The CRM system maintains all information in a single location that is always at your fingertips. These speeds up the procedure and boosts output.

7. Customer satisfaction rises when all consumers are efficiently attended to and given what they genuinely require. This increases the likelihood of acquiring more clients, which eventually boosts revenue and profit.

8. If a consumer is happy, they will always be loyal to you and will continue to use your services, which will build your customer base and ultimately boost your business's net growth.

9.1.11 Audit in Pharmacy

The audits are described as a "systematic, independent, and recorded procedure for acquiring audit evidence and objectively analysing it to ascertain the extent to which the verification criteria are met" by the International Organization for Standardization (ISO).In the pharmaceutical sector, audits serve as a virtual tool for determining whether established goals specified in the quality system are being met, creating the path for a continuous improvement program by giving management feedback. Audits are carried out to determine the accuracy and dependability of the data as well as to evaluate the internal control of a system. Simply said, an audit is the examination of a system or process to see whether it complies with the demands of its intended use.

Objective of audit

- Offering a chance for the quality management system to be improved.
- To evaluate whether the quality system is conforming to the required standards or not
- To examine the accuracy of the book of account.
- To express the view on the financial statement.
- Detection and prevention of frauds and errors.

Responsibility

1. An audit will assess the benefits and drawbacks of quality assurance and control procedures, and the findings will help us develop better procedures and systems for the benefit of the business.
2. Every pharmaceutical company's product contains features that need to be measured or validated by lab testing.
3. The necessary procedures that function as the control and balancing system in the pharmaceutical sector are quality control and quality assurance.

9.1.12   SOP of Pharmacy Management

A set of written instructions known as a standard operating procedure (SOP) describes the regularly recurring operations carried out by an institution. Sometimes the phrase "SOP" is used interchangeably with phrases like "protocols," "instructions," and "worksheets." A SOP is a requirement for learning. All changes in the instructions must be documented and reported to the authorities who are the only ones to authenticate and approve such variations.

Objectives of development of SOPS

- Elevate the level of service quality offered by the pharmacist.
- Encourage consistency in the services offered.
- Eliminate operational errors in pharmaceutical care delivery services.
- Promote the prestige of pharmacists and boost their drive for improved work.

- With SOPs in place, the pharmaceutical staff in a hospital may demonstrate that their operating procedures are secure and support continual improvement.

Importance of SOPS

Standard operating procedures are essential to maintain:

- Consistency - which helps to maintain the level of services offered and therefore maintains a good pharmaceutical practice at all times.
- Accuracy - to ensure that the services are offered with the highest level of attention, care, and due diligence to guarantee the safety of the patient and confidence of both the patient and the health worker.
- Reliability - this ensures that the outlined processes are dependable to achieve outcomes.
- Validity - to legalize processes within the pharmacy. People need consistency to achieve top performance and that is what SOPs provide. They reduce system variation, especially in systems where quality is very important e.g. manufacturing.

Benefits of SOPS

- SOPs provide benefits to the facility in different aspects and at the organizational level.
- SOPs help to assure the quality and consistency of medicine supply activities.
- People need consistency to achieve top performance.
- Productivity and performance are improved when jobs and tasks are done consistently.
- SOPs help staff to do that by giving clear instructions, which are available to all staff that does a certain task.
- The development and use of SOPs minimize variation and promote quality through the consistent implementation of a process or procedure within the organization, even if there are temporary or permanent personnel changes.
- SOPs provide an opportunity to fully utilize the expertise of all members of a department or team.
- People tend to be supportive of the things they help create. Involving employees in developing SOPs can help assure the final product is more complete, useful, and accepted.

- The SOP also helps senior managers to delegate responsibilities, and among staff, it assists in clarifying the roles of staff concerning specific tasks.

9.1.13 Introduction to Digital Health, mhealth, and Online Pharmacies

9.1.13.1 Digital health

In medicine and other health professions, the term "digital health" refers to the use of information and communication technologies to manage diseases, reduce health risks, and encourage wellness. The usage of wearable technology, mobile health, telehealth, health information technology, and telemedicine are all included in the vast field of digital health. Digital Health has been gaining momentum because it is envisioned to:

- Improve access to healthcare
- Reduce any inefficiencies in the healthcare system
- Improve the quality of care
- Lower the cost of healthcare
- Provide more personalized health care for patients

Categories of Digital Health Products and Services

1. Remote sensing and wearables
2. Telemedicine and health information
3. Data analytics and intelligence, predictive modelling
4. Bioinformatics tools (-omics)
5. Medical social media
6. Digitized health record platforms
7. Patient -physician-patient portals
8. DIY diagnostics, compliance, and treatments
9. Decision support systems

9.1.13.2 Mhealth

Pharmacists and patients have profited from the advancement of technology among healthcare practitioners globally. With these ongoing developments, pharmacists may enhance patient care by more effectively making information available and disseminating it. Due to financial constraints, geographic restrictions, labour shortages, and governance concerns, many low- and middle-income countries struggle to offer timely and effective healthcare. Mobile health is one method to overcome these challenges (mHealth). Utilizing mobile devices and other wireless technologies to deliver healthcare is known as mHealth. The World Health Organization (WHO) and the Global Observatory for eHealth have defined mHealth as "Medical and public health practice supported by mobile technologies, such as mobile phones, patient monitoring devices, personal digital assistants (PDAs), and other wireless devices. The term "health services and information offered or enhanced through the Internet and related technologies" is referred to as "eHealth," which is a large umbrella word.

9.1.13.3 Online pharmacy

Online pharmacies are places where customers can buy medications. They may also be referred to as virtual pharmacies, online pharmacies, or cyber pharmacies. The majority of online pharmacies acted only as a conduit between consumers and physical pharmacies. These businesses can be referred to as independent online pharmacies. For the expansion of their businesses, some physical pharmacies expand their service to the internet world. As they offer home delivery, convenient shopping, accessibility, a bigger selection, and a decrease in shopping time and effort, online pharmacies are becoming more and more popular every day. Refill reminder is a useful service provided by online pharmacies, in which the pharmacies notify customers when their prescriptions need to be filled again. For elderly patients or those with chronic diseases who must constantly purchase or replenish medications, they are very practical. Online pharmacies offer a huge selection of goods, such as over-the-counter (OTC) medications, prescription medications, medical equipment, pet medications, herbal products, and cosmetics.

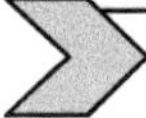 **Exercise Questions**

Multiple Choice Questions

1. The qualification for starting a retail sale drug store should be;
   a. Matriculate
   b. 10+2 with science
   c. Registered pharmacist
   d. D. pharmacy from unrecognised organization

2. Selection of site for a drug store is a:
   a. Significant decision   b. Insignificant decision
   c. Immaterial factor   d. All the above

3. Inventory includes
   a. Raw material, spar parts, maintaince, consumable goods
   b. Salaries of staff
   c. Assets and Liabilities
   d. Both 'a' an 'b'

4. A drug store is called an ideal drug store if its inventory is:
   a. Inadequate
   b. In excess
   c. In between minimum and maximum level
   d. None of the above

5. In VED analysis V stands for:
   a. Very good item   b. Very important item
   c. Vital items   d. Both 'a' and 'b'

Answers

1. c   2. a
3. d   4. c
5. c

Short Answer Questions

1. What is the purpose of ABC classification system?
2. What is general and restricted license?
3. Draw a layout of pharmacy store.
4. What is the characteristic of inventory control?
5. What is the characteristic of sound financial planning?
6. Explain day book with a table.
7. What is the importance of CRM?
8. What are the benefits of SOPs?
9. Why digital health product is ruling the market?
10. Elaborate online pharmacy.

Long Answer Questions

1. Explain in detail what are the legal requirement to set up the pharmacy store.
2. Describe the pharmacy design and its interior to run a successful pharmacy store.

3. What is inventory control and what are the different methods for inventory control?

4. Explain in detail financial planning. Why financial planning is important to run an organization.

5. What is cash book? Explain different types of cashbooks.